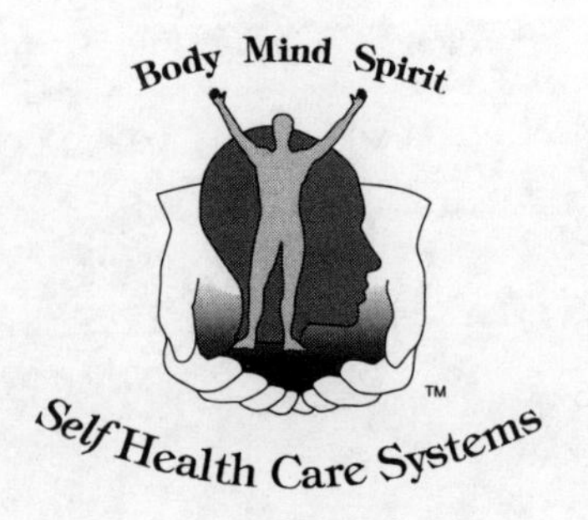
Body Mind Spirit
™
Self Health Care Systems

Awakening Our *Self*-Healing Body—

A Solution to the Health Care Crisis

Arthur M. Baker

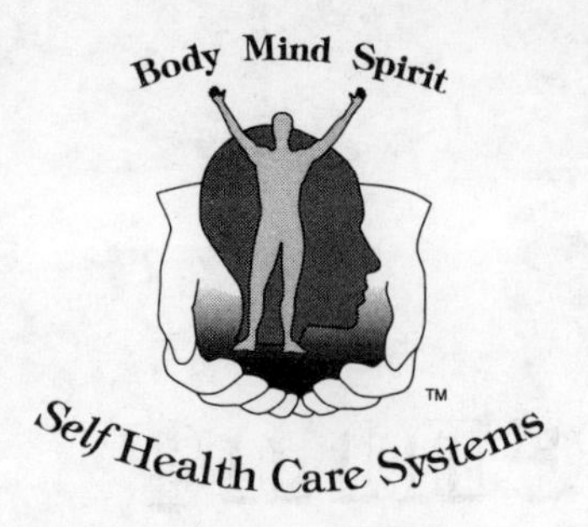

Published by:
Self Health Care Systems
1800 S. Robertson Blvd. Suite #239-1
Los Angeles CA. 90035

WARNING / DISCLAIMER

The author does not directly or indirectly dispense medical advise or prescribe the use of diet as a form of treatment for sickness without medical approval. Do not change your diet if you are seriously ill or on medication, except under the care of a medical doctor. Nutritionists and other experts in the field of health hold widely varying views. It is not the intent of the author to diagnose or prescribe. The intent is only to offer health information to help you cooperate with your doctor in your mutual quest for health. The information in this book is general, and not to be taken as professional advice for your specific health problems. Any decision you make involving the treatment of an illness should include the advice of the medical doctor of your choice. In the event you use this information without your doctor's approval, you are prescribing for yourself, which is your constitutional right, but the author and the publisher assume no responsibility.

Publishers--Cataloging in Publication
Baker, Arthur M.
Awakening our self-healing body--: a solution to the health care crisis / by Arthur M. Baker /
p. cm.
Includes bibliographical references and index.
Preassigned LCCN: 93-93516
ISBN 1-883989-25-6

1. Holistic medicine--United States. 2. Medical care--United States. I. Title

R733.B35 1993 610
QBI93-1035

About the Author

Unsatisfied with the status quo, Arthur M. Baker has always been an independent thinker in seeking out non-traditional means of education as an avenue to locate creative, innovative, yet practical solutions to problems of society.

He has been involved in the alternative health field for nearly 15 years, beginning in 1978 with studies that led to a B.A. in Natural Law (interdisciplinary science with an emphasis in biology) from Maharishi International University, Fairfield, Iowa.

Fully accredited by the Commission on Institutions of Higher Education of the North Central Association of Colleges and Schools, he also earned in 1986 an M.A. in Education from MIU, while studying the physiological relationships of human awareness to the physical body. At the same time, he acquired his secondary teaching credential from the Department of Public Instruction of the State of Iowa, where he has taught high school biology.

From 1986-1988, he studied health and nutritional science at the American College of Health Science (Life Science Institute), in Austin, Texas—the same institution that Harvey and Marilyn Diamond, the authors of *Fit For Life*, attended.

Currently, he is president of Self-Health Care Systems, a health education and consulting service (located at 1800 S. Robertson Blvd., Suite #239-1 Los Angeles, CA 90035), and teaches health and science in the Los Angeles public schools. Mr. Baker lectures and gives seminars on health related educational issues, and he is finishing his second book which addresses the non-viral causes of AIDS.

This book is dedicated to all those who are sincerely seeking health—who, chances are, have been exploited to some degree by those selling drugs, potions, magical therapies, and various exotic "cures."

Acknowledgements

I would like to thank Judy and Daisy for listening, for their patience, and for their continual feedback; Terry Monika for his tedious detail; Mohammad and Linda at Printex; Steven Grossinger, Jim Seavall at Personal Support Computers, Todd Meisler at RPI, Larry Davis at Griffin Printing, and Laura Leimseider (photographer); and the Atman for guidance. Foremost, MMY and JGD.

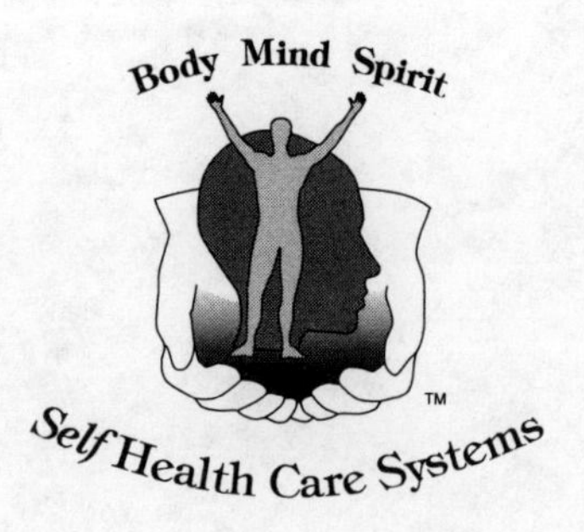
Body Mind Spirit
Self Health Care Systems
TM

Table of Contents

Section III
The Solution in Theory and Practice: Natural Hygiene—the True Self Health Care System

Section IV
Let's Get Technical: The "Nuts and Bolts" of the Self-Healing Body—Why Self-Health Care Works

Section V
But How About Bacteria, Germs, and Viruses—Aren't They the Cause of Disease?

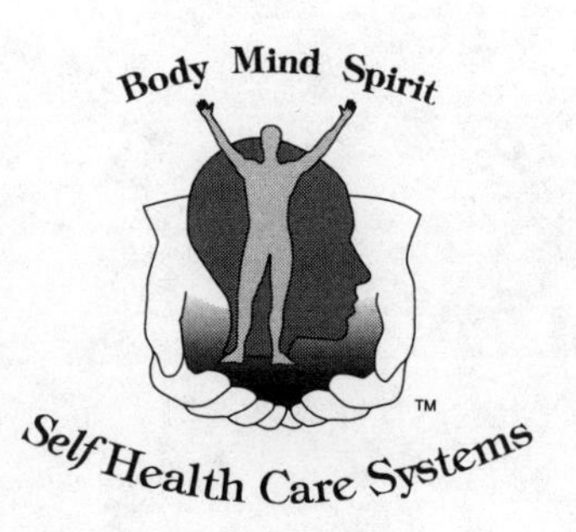
Body Mind Spirit
Self Health Care Systems

Introduction

If there is one thing agreed upon by "experts" and lay people in this country regarding health care, it is that the system works poorly, it is wasteful, and needs drastic, not merely cosmetic, reform.

This is a book about health reform. Interestingly, the word "reform" is defined as follows: to correct errors and abuses; to make more just, or humane; to improve in form, style and method; and to give up evil ways. Although I would not go so far as to call our U.S. health care system evil, it definitely is a seriously flawed, poorly managed, error ridden system—whose very theoretical basis in its approach to health needs to be adjusted to make it more humane.

The focus of health care into the next century needs to be placed on educating the public on the genuine biological needs of the human body. Western medicine does not study health; rather, it studies disease. The Western approach to health care, called ***allopathic*** medicine, treats symptoms with drugs and does not teach the public the essentials of health that are required to build and maintain a vibrant state of well-being.

It must be understood that when I speak of health, I do not mean merely a lack of illness, nor am I referring to the ordinary low levels of energy usually experienced by the majority of Americans—many of whom drag themselves out of bed each morning and whip their physiology with doses of caffeine and/or nicotine in preparation for yet another draining day.

Instead, when I speak of health, I mean not only physical wellness where the body functions smoothly and efficiently into old age, but an attitude whereby we start each day with the energy and enthusiasm to meet our daily challenges with courage and confidence. **To achieve such a state of health is a matter of skill not luck or "good genes."** Skill is based on education. We must be taught not only the requirements of health, but also what harmful substances and influences to avoid.

There is *so much* confusing and conflicting "health" information on the market today, that people are frustrated—and I cannot blame them. Unfortunately, almost everything in the media regarding health represents a vested interest selling some sort of drug, pill, potion, high-tech treatment or therapy, rather than providing viable, practical, reliable and easily understood information on true health education. And there is reason for this.

If the public were healthy, there would be no need for medicines, herbs and treatments. What is known as "health care" in this country, whether traditional or "alternative," has a vested interest in illness, not wellness and, therefore, may be more accurately described as "disease care."

Without sickness, business is slow. While there are sincere individuals in the health care field working diligently to decrease suffering, efforts would pay off much more if energy and resources were redirected to teaching self-sufficiency in matters of health care—the very purpose of this book.

The body is an automatically self-healing organism, for this is programmed into the very genetic blueprint of life. Due to constant unhealthful obstacles provided by our daily insalubrious lifestyle (to which we are not biologically adapted), our bodies become diseased and age prematurely.

We need to learn how to awaken our self-healing body by providing the optimal conditions for health to re-establish itself. The implementation of this strategy, and its theoretical basis, embodies a major portion of this book.

The first section looks in detail at the problem—our ailing health care system. The next two sections focus on the solution—health reform based on our biological adaptations and how physiology operates

The theory and practical application of holistic self-health care is also discussed in detail. This is followed by section four, which covers the technical aspects of the self-healing body and the specifics of why self-health care works. Section five dispels medical myths regarding bacteria, germs and viruses as the causes of disease. The last section inspires those who sincerely desire health to create it—through proper lifestyle.

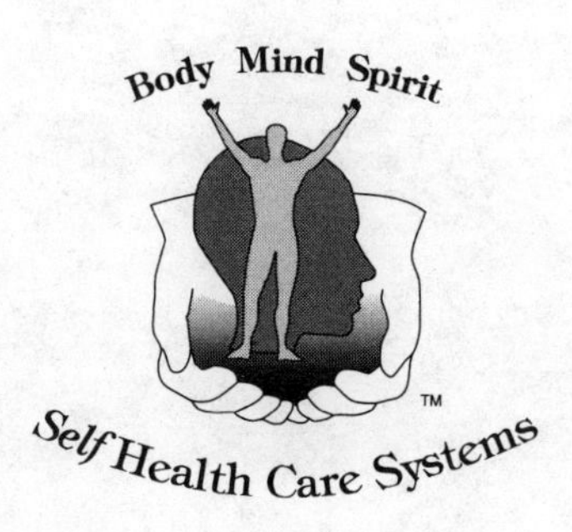
Body Mind Spirit
TM
Self Health Care Systems

SECTION I

THE PROBLEM:

OUR AILING HEALTH CARE SYSTEM

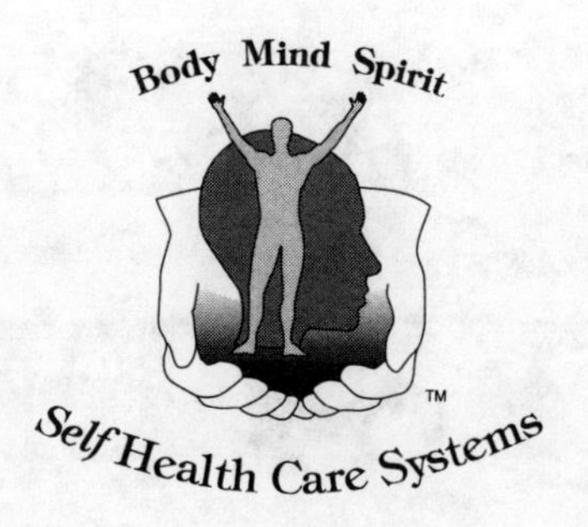
Body Mind Spirit
Self Health Care Systems
TM

Chapter 1

HEALTH CARE IS BANKRUPTING AMERICA AND LEAVING US INCREASINGLY DISEASED

Nearly every newspaper, magazine, television and radio news program has weekly if not daily reports on the current health care crisis in our country. Alarming quotes from experts and information from government sources command attention to the problem and demand immediate action to stem the crisis.

For example:

- Former Surgeon General Everett Koop has said "Our health care system is in crisis, bordering on chaos";
- Dr. Philip Caper, medical policy analyst at Dartmouth Medical School states "I can't imagine a system that's more dysfunctional than the one we have now—more expensive, not doing the job, with more waste"; and
- according to Prof. E. Cheraskin M.D., of the University of Alabama School of Medicine, "health is the largest failing business in America".

There are three separate health care problems in the United States, and each is at odds with the other:

1. Costs are exploding;
2. Thirty seven million Americans lack health insurance; and
3. Our present system of "health care" may be more accurately described as "disease care" since it is leaving us ever more sick and diseased.

To comprehend the magnitude of the health care crisis, each of these problems needs to be understood separately, as well as how they interrelate.

The depressed economy, increasing unemployment and lack of growth has contributed dramatically to the growing concern about health care. Between 1989 and 1990, the yearly burden on American families to pay for health care increased to over $6,500, of which $4,300 is actually paid by families and the rest by businesses. Of this $4,300, 32% comes *directly* out of the pocket; 40% from general taxes; 17% goes towards insurance premiums and the remaining 11% is paid by Medicare —and this isn't just Monopoly money.

All health care dollars come out of household budgets directly through taxes, insurance premiums, higher prices for products and services, and from lower wages. Americans without health insurance are forced to forgo treatment or are crowded into emergency rooms with waiting times reminiscent of Russian bread lines. For would-be health reformers, the challenge is to control costs, simultaneously expand access, while still ensuring "quality care."

The health care crisis is distorting the shape of our economy and is slowly bankrupting America. While the national medical bill for 1992 rang in at over $817 billion, the bill for 1993 stands at $912 billion.

The Commerce department reports that health care costs are climbing at a pace four times higher than the rate of overall inflation. The total cost of health care which was expected to top $1 trillion by the turn of the century seems likely to hit that level by 1994-1995. Spending has been projected at more than $1.4 trillion by the year 2000, and close to $2 trillion by the year 2002. If this same rate of growth continues unabated, health care spending will very soon reach unsustainable levels.

Americans now spend over $25,000 a second, and over $2 billion per day each year on health care. A mere 1% of the population accounts for 29% of all medical costs, while 5% are responsible for half the total—yet the way our current health insurance system is structured, nearly EVERYONE gets stuck splitting the bill.

James C. Robinson, health care economist at the University of California, Berkeley, explains the problem this way: "Imagine if we sold auto-purchase insurance and said go and buy whatever car you want and we'll pay 80% of it." Under those conditions, many people would buy a Mercedes. If nothing is done to stem the tide, the average family's outlay for health care will double by the end of the decade from about $4,300 per year to about $9,400 annually.

In an article from the April 17, 1993 edition of the Los

Angeles Times entitled "First Lady Issues Warning on Health Care," Hillary Clinton warns that without sweeping changes in health care reform, increases in costs will plague many Americans. Local and state governments also risk bankruptcy due to potentially ruinous cost increases.

If we do nothing to stem the tide, she warned, health care costs will more than double in the next few years, and the average family will be paying some $14,000 per year in insurance premiums, out-of-pocket costs, and in health care related taxes.

Health care costs have spiraled out of control. Costs consume about 16% of state and local tax revenues and since 1986, private businesses have spent as much on health care as they earned in after-tax profits. For small businesses, health insurance is unaffordable. Three of every four companies who employ 10 people or less do not provide any health benefits. This is a major contributing factor in the fact that roughly 37 million Americans have no health coverage whatsoever.

Large employers and corporations who provide coverage for 85% of their workers are staggering under the costs of health care. Among the hardest hit are industrial giants which support millions of elderly retirees whose medical bills far exceed younger employees.

Under the burden, Ford Motor Company wrote-off $7.5 billion in their fourth quarter of 1992 to account for health care costs of retirees, a blow that will probably force Ford to report the largest annual loss ever by a U.S. Corporation—nearly $7 billion. AT&T expects to take a similar write-off this year, and General Motors, with far more retirees, faces a similar catastrophic deficit when it too takes the health care hit.

And the problem is not only sky-rocketing costs. A growing number of employers have stopped providing insurance to workers. *Each month* , about 100,000 Americans join the growing rolls of those lacking health care insurance.

Nearly 100 Million Americans Are Uninsured or Underinsured

America is the only industrialized nation in the world that does not guarantee medical care for its citizens. Between 1989 and 1990, the number of uninsured and those underinsured grew dramatically as companies cut back or continuously eliminated benefits. During this same time frame, 1.3 million additional Americans were added to the list of those without coverage, of whom 74% earned more than $25,000 annually.

In total, over 37 million Americans are uninsured and an additional 50 million to 60 million are underinsured. These individuals hold bare bones coverage with major restrictions or completely uncovered services.

Ironically, more than half of those who are uninsured work full time and pay taxes that support government subsidized health insurance programs for the poor, the elderly, and for veterans. The problem is high cost. Medical insurance premiums cost the average American about $5,600 each year.

In a report by the Families USA Foundation, 46% of U.S. families in 1993 have at least one member who either will have no health insurance or who will spend 10% OR MORE of his or her personal income to pay medical bills. In total, 25 million Americans will be paying out-of-pocket medical expenses which do not include Medicare payroll tax deductions, or other state, federal, and local taxes that pay for health care.

Most hard hit are the elderly since Medicare often does not cover costs for prescriptions or long term home-delivered health care. *And neither do the supplemental policies that are often purchased supposedly to fill in the gaps in their Medicare coverage.*

Families USA, a nationwide health care consumer group which influences policy within the Clinton Administration, based its study on national statistics gathered by federal agencies. According to its report, 57.3 million Americans will be without health insurance sometime during 1993 because of changing jobs or changes in coverage—a figure much higher than previous estimates.

If criminals have the fundamental right in this country to a lawyer, then working Americans should have the right to health care if the need arises, including preventive care. Sixty percent of all poor people are not even covered by Medicaid and only one million of 30 million senior citizens have long-term health care coverage. In 1990, almost one quarter of pregnant American women received no prenatal care—a figure that has risen 50% since the Reagan Administration of the 1980s.

Mental-health services in this country are even more abominable. In 1991, the National Mental Health Association reported that of the 153 million Americans with private health insurance coverage, the accessibility to mental health services is *much more* restrictive than are physical health services—benefits are far less comprehensive; maximum benefits are substantially lower; deductibles higher; and the percentage reimbursed significantly smaller.

U.S. Health Care Leaves us Diseased

If our current health care system was worth the price in producing results—making us healthier than those elsewhere, it might be worth it. But of the 24 industrialized nations that comprise the Organization for Economic Cooperation and Development (OECD), **the U.S. spends twice as much on health care than anywhere worldwide** even though all OECD countries, except for Turkey and Greece (which are by far the poorest), all have about the same number of doctors and hospitals per capita as our country. As far as health status among the 24 OECD countries, the U.S. ranks as follows:

- 21st in infant mortality;
- 17th in male life expectancy; and
- 16th in female life expectancy.

In nearly all areas, the U.S. ranks at or near the bottom.

Health care in this country is the most expensive in the world, yet 15 countries outrank our nation in life expectancy. While U.S. expenditures are nearly double Japan's and Switzerland's as a percentage of its Gross Domestic Product (GDP) for example, U.S. life expectancy is significantly lower than both of these two countries as listed below:

- 71.6 years for American men;
- 78.6 years for American women;
- 74.1 years for Swiss men;
- 81.3 years for Swiss women;
- 76.2 years for Japanese men; and
- 82.5 years for Japanese women.

Comparing U.S. health care to other nations, it is clear that people elsewhere pay less, are healthier, and live longer lives. ***In Canada, the national health care budget is 40% less than ours and in most Europeon countries 50% less while each produces healthier citizens and, hence, better quality health care.*** Costs are kept down by eliminating waste; expensive equipment is shared between hospitals; and fees for medical procedures are well-defined.

Alan Sager, health economist at Boston University School of Public Health says "look at the rest of the industrialized world. On the average, they spend half as much as we do on health care. They cover everyone and live longer. It's waste. There's no other explanation."

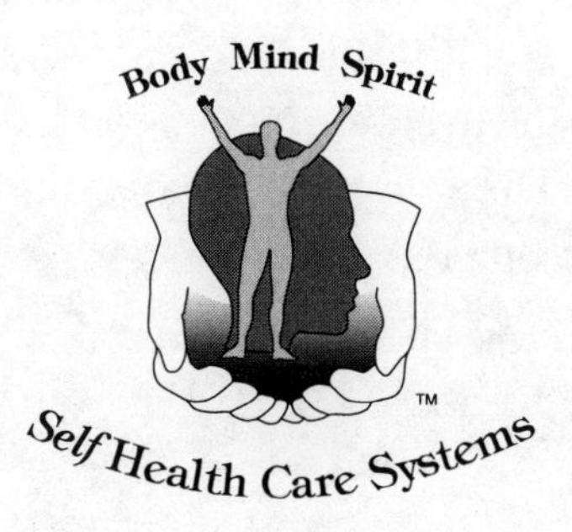
Body Mind Spirit
TM
Self Health Care Systems

Chapter 2

HIGH PRICES, HIGH PROFITS, AND OUR WASTED HEALTH CARE DOLLARS— AND THERE'S NO CONTROLLING THE COSTS

Our health care system is rigged such that it DEMANDS that prices constantly rise. The system allows doctors to order whatever procedures they want and pays physicians and hospitals whatever they think they should get. In both respects, the American system stands alone in the developed world.

Canada, Japan, and Western Europeon countries have adopted universal standard payment schedules set by direct negotiation with doctors and hospitals. Most have also set a ceiling on national medical expenditures. As a result, only the U.S. devoted more than 10% of its GDP to health care—and we broke that barrier in 1985.

In 1992, 14% of our GDP was spent on health care and according to projections, by the year 2030, health care costs could reach 25% of our GDP. To put this into perspective, the U.S. spends just under six percent of its GDP on education and about the same on national defense. Health care outlays however, account for more of the GDP than these two *combined.*

Back in 1960, however, our nation spent a modest 5.3% of its GDP on health care, about the same as Canada, Germany, and other industrialized countries at that time. The advent of Medicare in 1965 changed everything dramatically. Before then, most insured individuals had only hospital coverage, and no insurance to cover doctor bills. Physicians, therefore, tended to keep fees affordable. In 1965, the government financed health insurance for the elderly via Medicare, as well as with Medicaid, where costs were shared with the individual states.

In order to overcome the powerful political opposition of doctors and hospitals to "socialized" medicine, Congress made the expensive mistake of allowing doctors to be paid on the basis of their "usual and customary" fees (the system Blue Shield was already using). This allowed physicians to name their own price without constraints on costs. Predictably, doctor fees soared.

Hospitals also greatly profited. Under Medicare, not only were they allowed to collect actual charges for tests, supplies, services, etc., but for the first time they were allowed to add the cost of capital improvements into their rates which gave them further federally subsidized incentive to rapidly expand.

Pharmaceutical companies and manufacturers of medical

equipment have also profited massively over the recent years. They charge top dollar for their products, secure in knowing the system will reimburse them. The drug industry is one of the nations' most profitable—operating with an average 15% profit margin and giving back an average annual return of 25% to investors over the last decade.

Americans pay more for medicine than virtually anyone else worldwide. According to a 1992 survey released by the General Accounting Office (the investigating arm of Congress), prescription drugs cost an average of 32% more in the U.S. than in Canada. For the 200 best selling drugs, prices charged by pharmacies rose 6.4% last year compared to a 1.5% increase for all other finished goods.

This has made the $55 billion pharmaceutical industry the nation's most profitable business. Among the Fortune 500 drug companies, the median return on investment for drug manufacturers averages 26%—twice the average for all other Fortune 500 industries. **Health care stocks as a group increased in value by over 50% in 1991.** The bottom line is that a lot of people in health care are cashing in and they're not unhappy with the current system.

In 1990, for instance, hospitals soaked up 38% of national health expenditures (twice as much as doctors) while earning a profit of $7 billion. William Erwin, spokesman for the American Hospital Association explains "hospitals make money by delivering services. If you don't need much done to you, the hospital isn't going to make money."

While individual doctors have great leeway in deciding their charge for a given procedure, insurance companies use computer data banks to determine whether the fee is "usual and customary." Fees at the top of the scale may not receive full reimbursement. But in the case of new procedures, there's no such track record and price is set accordingly, *which rarely comes down after the procedure becomes routine* .

In the early 1980s for example, cataract extraction and artificial lens implantation was introduced and became a standard procedure by the end of the decade. Opthalmologists during that time became wealthy charging $2,000 or more for cataract extraction performed in about an hour.

And There's No Controlling the Costs

Over the last ten years as medical costs have become truly staggering, the system has tried to change but to no avail. Medicare has set limits on physician fees, and Medicaid budgets have been cut back to the point where many states now pay doctors and hospitals less than the cost of delivering care.

But experience has shown that attempts to manage the health care system in a piecemeal manner are likely to fail. Physicians and hospitals charge their privately insured patients more money to make-up for Medicare fee restrictions. In 1986, in the midst of a Medicare freeze on physician fees, doctors increased their services and collected 15% more from Medicare then they had the previous year.

In the April 1, 1993 edition of the Los Angeles Times, it is reported that market experts and economists warn of the Clinton Administration's proposed health care price controls actually *backfiring* and INCREASING costs in the long run.

Price controls did not work for the Carter, Nixon, or Franklin D. Roosevelt Administrations, and some Clinton advisors are suggesting that any attempt to use them now will also likely meet with failure since such efforts would lead to massive evasion of the rules, and to bureaucratic chaos throughout the health care industry.

Without price controls, Vice President Al Gore says that health care costs will rise from 14% to 20% of the GDP by the year 2000. Ira Magaziner, the chief health care advisor for the Clinton Administration, adds that without price controls, health care costs will grow 11% a year.

Three means of controlling prices are being considered: an outright freeze on all prices at existing levels; a cap on insurance premiums combined with a rule prohibiting cuts in benefits; and legislation forcing insurers to charge all patients the same fees they now receive from the government for treating Medicare patients.

Economists warn that an outright freeze on all health care prices would require a massive government bureaucracy in order to regulate the one-seventh of the American economy that such legislation would effect. Similarly, economists argue that Medicare reimbursement rates are artificial and bear no relation to actual costs—and that caps on insurance premiums will drive some insurers either into bankruptcy or out of business altogether.

Economists predict that if the government gets involved in setting fees for doctor's office visits, they will simply require patients to make more appointments, thereby defeating the very purpose of price controls; and if the government sets prices for drugs, pharmaceutical companies will slightly modify their products to justify increasing their prices.

One solution for physicians is to require them to publicly disclose their fees, thereby encouraging patients to shop around since most have no idea what they will be charged before visiting a doctor.

But according to Barry Bosworth, who was in charge of President Carter's failed effort to restrain prices, "the health care industry is the best example of an industry where price controls won't work." Echoing these remarks, C. Jackson Gray who chaired Nixon's price commission in the early 1970s said "price controls will make things worse."

History demonstrates that price controls are ineffective in

restraining inflation; are not easily enforced; require unwieldy government bureaucracy; and end up distorting markets they are intended to control. On the contrary, they are actually *blamed* for fueling inflation rather than restraining it.

Despite the unpromising history of price controls, opinion polls show that Americans favor imposing fee restraints on doctors, insurance carriers, and pharmaceutical companies. Clinton is considering price controls because he sees no other way, in the short term (other than raising taxes), to fund the $50 billion to $90 billion per year required to finance health insurance coverage for all Americans.

Medical System Takes Healthy Care of its Bottom Line

Having operated for years under a system that set no limit on charges, doctors and patients have been brainwashed to believe that in treating sickness, EVERYTHING must be done—more procedures, more tests, more pills, and more time with the doctor.

Says Randall Bovbjerb, health policy analyst at the Urban Institute in Washington D.C., "We can't sit and watch the course of a cold, we go and buy tons of things we aren't even certain will make it better."

Our health system is geared to provide services that earn physicians and hospitals the most money—not those that provide the most care to the public.

The U.S., for example, has four times the Magnetic Resonance Imaging (MRI) devices per capita (costing $1.5 million each) than does Germany. At the same time, however, the U.S. system shortchanges the poor and uninsured.

In the 1980s, while hospitals were adding costly high-tech equipment at a furious clip, the number of pregnant mothers unable to get prenatal care climbed, as did the rate of premature births. In most states, Medicaid pays nowhere near the actual cost of delivery, and public hospitals lose money. As a result, many doctors and for-profit hospitals refuse Medicaid patients.

American physicians are heavy purveyors of expensive treatments and diagnostic tests—and reap great financial rewards for using them.

According to figures from the Organization for Economic Cooperation and Development, in 1987 U.S. doctors earned 5.4 times more than the average U.S. worker; in Germany doctors earned 4.2 times more than German workers; Canada 3.7 times; and France, Japan, and the U.K., 2.4 times their citizens.

How rich are doctors? Over the past decade, physicians have significantly widened their income over the general population.

Whereas full time male workers in this country average about $32,000, and females just over $20,000, physicians average $130,000 annually. Surgeons and radiologists make over $200,000; cardiovascular surgeons in group practice, $500,000; gynecologists, over $180,000; pediatricians, $100,000; and family practitioners, $93,000 annually.

There is no doubt that the American health care system is currently on the operating table, with doctors themselves under the knife. While critics hold physicians largely responsible for runaway costs, consumer advocate Ron Pollack of Families USA explains: "I don't think the American public can have a great deal of sympathy for incomes that are six times what the average worker receives, and rising at rates far in excess of what other workers are receiving."

Interestingly, when physicians explain why health care costs continually rise, they frequently respond with complaints regarding malpractice that "encourages unnecessary defensive medical care", and the public tends to believe this argument without question.

According to Medical Economics magazine, however, in

1990 doctor's malpractice premiums on average consumed only 3.7% of their receipts. The U.S. Department of Health and Human Services puts the total cost of malpractice at less than 1% of total health outlays.

Fraud and Outright Waste

The more procedures doctors perform under our current system of health care, the more they get paid—a situation guaranteed to cause costs to surge out of control. Business volume increases dramatically with a few more tests, schedule a few more doctor visits, and reduce the time spent on each visit.

The creation of medical "need" by those who profit from it is called *induced demand* and it runs rampant, especially where physicians refer patients for treatment to facilities where they have a financial interest.

Consider MRI (Magnetic Resonance Imaging devices)—a powerful new imaging technique that produces detailed pictures of internal organs without radiation exposure. The procedure costs $1,000 a shot (versus $177 in Japan for the same procedure) and some U.S. physicians who invest in MRI profit by unnecessarily referring their patients for the test. Experts stress that MRI should be ordered only when diagnosis cannot be determined any other way.

Since the mid-1980s, doctors have also been manipulating the reimbursement system by "unbundling" services—charging for separate component procedures instead of the one that was actually performed. For example, rather than billing $1,200 for a hysterectomy, doctors can collect $7,000 by billing separately for the individual procedures that make-up the operation.

Commercial services conduct seminars counseling doctors how to maximize reimbursements this way, but unbundling can quickly become fraudulent. In addition, dishonest physicians cheat insurance companies by billing for more office visits than can reasonably be performed in a single day—which may not be detected when billing is spread among numerous insurance payers.

U.S. health care is obsessed with making sure patients get only what their insurance entitles them to and nothing more. Hospitals must keep meticulous records of every patient, down to individual gauze bandages and aspirin tablets—all of which adds to administrative costs.

Dealing with the multitude of insurance forms requires an army of clerical power to the tune of a whopping 20% of U.S. hospital operating budgets, compared to 9% in Canadian hospitals.

To operate a health plan covering 25 million citizens, Canada employs fewer administrators than Massachusetts Blue Cross which covers 2.7 million citizens. In total, about 20% of U.S. health care costs go toward administration and billing expenses, compared to about 10% in the Canadian single-payer system.

In 1991, the General Accounting Office, estimated that a shift to a single-payer health care system would cut overhead costs $34 billion annually by decreasing repetitive paperwork and administrative procedures. By standardizing the more than 1,500 different insurance forms currently in use, wasteful billing costs could be reduced dramatically.

According to Consumer Reports (July 1992) in an article entitled "Wasted Health Care Dollars", of the $817 billion spent in 1992 on health care, AT LEAST $200 billion is thrown away on a huge bureaucracy that sucks up over $100 billion per year alone, and on overpriced, useless, and even harmful medical treatments.

After extensive review of the literature, researchers believe that $200 billion is a *conservative* estimate of the waste in 1992 health care costs. Of the $817 billion spent on health care, a full one-fifth ($163 billion) went for administrative costs alone. Except for a fraction of a percent spent on research, the remaining $650 billion went to actual patient care—of which AT LEAST 20% ($130 billion) was spent on clearly unnecessary procedures, services, and hospital stays.

Most notable among medical treatments that are overused and frequently unnecessary are caesarean sections, hysterectomies, back surgeries, and Magnetic Resonance Imaging (MRI) just to name a few.

One in four births in this country is completed surgically—making caesarean sections the number one major surgery in this country. This rate is estimated to be twice the amount necessary. Hospitals that have systematically eliminated unnecessary caesarean sections have cut their rate AT LEAST in half without risk to mothers or babies (see *Consumer Reports*, February 1991).

After caesarean sections, hysterectomies are the second most common major surgery in this country. Value Health Service, using methodologies developed by Rand, calls 27% of hysterectomies unnecessary. Likewise, it reports that back surgery (laminectomy) is unnecessary 14% of the time.

Other unnecessary procedures include 27% of surgeries for Carpal Tunnel Syndrome (an uncomfortable wrist ailment); 16% for tonsillectomies; 60% of pre-operative laboratory screening procedures; and 30% of upper gastrointestinal X-ray tests.

Again according to Consumer Reports, if overuse of medical services wastes $130 billion annually, administrative inefficiency adds about $70 billion.

Projections from 1991 estimates of the General Accounting Office indicate the U.S. could save about $70 billion each year by switching from the current fragmented and inefficient multi-insurance system to a single-payer system, where a single insurance entity pays private doctors and hospitals for services rendered to the individual.

Savings would come from insurance company overhead, and hospital, and administrative costs—and at least 20% of the money now spent on health care in this country could be saved with no loss in the quality of medical care. Easily, there is more than enough excess spending in our health care system to cover the roughly 14% of the population not currently under any insurance plan.

Adding the $130 billion figure to the $70 billion gives an estimate of $200 billion annual waste in our current health care system. This conservative figure, however, leaves out several important elements that could potentially blow this $200 billion estimate sky-high. For example:

1. Physicians' fees, costs of drugs, procedures, and medical technology—if these costs were brought into line with standards in other industrialized countries, the annual savings would be significantly greater.

2. The cost of outright fraud has not been calculated into this figure, a factor the General Accounting Office estimates could swallow a full 10% of the total health care budget (nearly $82 billion).

For instance, some physicians cheat the system by ordering unnecessary tests and procedures; some bill for services never rendered; some falsify reimbursement codes to collect more money than is actually due; and some submit inflated bills for supplies and medical devices.

On March 3, 1993, the Los Angeles Times reported on the biggest case of health care fraud in U.S. history where two brothers, Michael and David Smushkevich, ripped off health insurance companies and the U.S. government to the tune of $1 billion.

By using telemarketing pitches and advertisements to lure patients with offers of free physicals to a vast network of clinics throughout Southern California, the brothers put patients through unneeded high-tech tests and charged insurance companies an average of $8,000 per person.

Taxpayer-funded military insurance plans were also defrauded, as the enterprise allegedly billed over twice what the entire state of California spends on medical care for indigent patients each year. Even though patients were entirely healthy, the Smushkevich's would falsify paperwork to justify insurance billings by claiming that patients had serious health problems including cancer and heart disease.

In this way, thousands of healthy individuals were turned into sickly cash cows on paper alone. Despite the arrests, insurance companies are currently tracking hundreds of spinoff-copycat operations that are still running rolling labs in California and across the country.

Including cases such as these, it is estimated that U.S. health care dollars are wasted as follows:

1. ***Pure fraud*:** approximately $70 billion;
2. ***Semi-fraud and unnecessary treatments*:** $100 billion-$130 billion;
3. ***Bureaucracy***: $50 billion-$70 billion; and
4. ***Overpricing and lack of cost management***: $60 billion-$80 billion.

Chapter 3

PLAYING POLITICS WITH U.S. HEALTH CARE

With all the problems plaguing U.S. health care, what *does* prevent our country from adopting a rational, humane health care system? Several assumptions, including every advance in medicine must immediately be adopted regardless of cost, effectiveness, or duplication; expectations of huge incomes for most physicians; and that the role of government is to enhance profits and to protect the status quo.

The cost of health care in this country has reached such a magnitude, however, that it is now politically impossible to ignore—especially in the light of its declining effectiveness as measured by infant mortality and life expectancy rates and the tens of millions of Americans who are entirely shut out of the system due to no health insurance whatsoever.

And YOU Will Pay With Higher Taxes

The Los Angeles Times, on March 18 and March 23, 1993, reported that government spending on medical bills for the nation's poor soared 25% last year, which illustrates once more, the extreme difficulties the Clinton Administration faces in its efforts to control health care costs.

President Clinton has promised to provide universal coverage including health insurance, for 37 million Americans who live without it—a pledge that will cost from $50 billion to $90 billion a year. It is unclear how this will be accomplished without substantial tax increases.

In the May 1 and May 7, 1993 editions of the Los Angeles Times, two articles entitled "New Payroll Deduction May Fund Health Plan," and "Payroll Levy Idea in Health Plan Detailed" describe how the Clinton Administration is seeking a *new* payroll deduction similar to the taxes already being exhumed regularly from paychecks for Social Security, Medicare, and disability insurance, to pay for health care reform.

To finance health care reform, the government is considering *mandatory* payroll deductions as high as 7% for companies and 2-3% for workers. Such a levy would be in addition to deductions of 7.65% currently taken from workers' paychecks for Social Security and Medicare, and matched by employers. The new tax would allow businesses to stop directly paying insurance companies for covering their workers.

The broad health care payroll deduction would be based on the percentage of income earned and would hit hard at highly compensated workers, who typically pay out-of-pocket costs of much less than 2-3% of their income for medical coverage. Similarly, a 7% payroll tax would be a huge blow to small businesses, many of whom do not offer medical insurance to their workers. Corporate America would benefit, however—

especially the manufacturing giants with an aging work force, such as auto companies, who now pay 14% or more of their payroll for employee health benefits.

Currently, payroll taxes total 15.3%—split evenly between the employer and the worker. The deductions for workers include 6.2% for Social Security, and 1.45% for Medicare. It is unclear whether the proposed new payroll tax, if adopted by Congress, would be sufficient to finance the overall health care reforms planned by President Clinton.

Health Care analysts explain that a 9-10% payroll levy could raise about $300 billion a year, but this would be offset by the estimated $200 billion now spent by employers for workers' health benefits, and the estimated $55 billion being spent by employees themselves—most of which would cease, due to insurance companies no longer being *directly* paid by employers if the new payroll levy plan is implemented.

In some shape or form, the Clinton Administration, in order to pay for health care reform, IS RAISING TAXES nearly across the board. Rather than cut out waste and redirect the savings, more of our dollar will be taxed and fed into a seriously flawed system.

Also, as reported in the April 9, 1993 edition of the Los Angeles Times rising health care costs in this country may totally erase attempts by President Clinton to make significant cuts in the federal deficit. Despite all the proposed tax increases, and despite the large cuts in national defense spending, Clinton's proposed budget would produce only moderate improvements in the long standing federal deficit due to the constantly climbing costs of federal health care programs.

In 1993, Medicare, Medicaid, and other federal health programs will cost $244 billion TAX dollars, accounting for 16% of every federal dollar. In 1998, however, the bill for these health care programs is projected to rise to just below $400 billion, or 22% of each tax dollar. Leon E. Ponetta, director of the White House Office of Management and Budget, said if these trends continue, health care costs would "triple as we enter the next century, almost quadruple."

Spending is increasing due to several factors:

1. Medicaid spending, the joint state-federal program that covers costs for the poor, has sharply increased because of more poor people due to the recession;
2. Congress has expanded eligibility to Medicaid to include more poor pregnant woman;
3. Medicare, the federal health insurance program for the elderly has grown as has the age of the country's seniors; and
4. The overall high rate of inflation and uncontrolled price increases in the health care field. The impact of these soaring costs on both the federal budget and on the private sector has created the crisis fueling Clinton's drive to reform the nation's health care system.

Due to soaring, ever-escalating health care costs, Clinton's budget planners project the federal deficit will continue to rise after just a few years following only short initial gains made from improvements in the economy and from a sobering dose of new taxes. Unless these costs are brought permanently under control, *all* of the Administration's deficit reductions will be entirely wiped out shortly after the year 2000.

Radical change is necessary—including a new fundamental understanding of what actual health care must entail—if a truly viable model is to be implemented that will generate massive improvement in our nation's health. Whatever type of health care reform is implemented, it is clear that it must be radically different from the wasteful profit-oriented framework that currently governs our medical system.

The U.S. health care system is bleeding money and it requires an immediate tourniquet followed by a thorough purification program. Wasteful treatments, unlimited access to our choice of doctors, and the highest-priced technology must be forgone to stanch the problem. **The public is now beginning to inquire not merely how to get well but how to STAY well.**

Drastically reducing health care costs in this country not only would improve health but would also help our debt-ridden country get back on the right course. In order for this to occur, special interest groups who influence our elected representatives through various financial contributions and outright (although legal) bribes must be removed from government.

Ideas introduced by Bush and Clinton on health care have never been carried out because they would offend one or more powerful special interest groups including drug companies, insurance carriers, doctors, and even patients.

Five key special interest groups and what they want out of health care reform are summarized below:

1. **Doctors** oppose price controls and rigid national budgets that impose penalties for exceeding spending above pre-set levels. Instead, physicians want a system that preserves the patient's choice of which doctor they wish to see and one that permits a fee-for-service option.
2. **Hospitals** oppose extension of the Medicare payment system to everyone and are against altering fees or reimbursement schedules without restructuring these to involve doctors.
3. **Drug Companies** oppose mandatory price controls; favor voluntary price-increase restraints. They also want to see drug coverage as part of the overall program of health care benefits.
4. **Insurance Companies** oppose plans that mandate a single regional purchaser of health insurance; they are also against premium caps.
5. **Patients** oppose any plan that would limit the right to choose their own doctor.

Any interest group hit by the president's plan for health care reform will charge that "reform" is a code word for *less* health care than the middle class is now getting under the current system.

The right to choose your own doctor could be pitted against any plan that will inevitably restrict choice in the name of curbing health care costs by rationing—made necessary by greedy doctors and insurance companies. Under the current health care system, there already is no choice of doctors for a huge chunk of the population, while rationing is dictated by the ability to pay.

But shouldn't the real question here be the right to choose between a true "health-care" system that *educates* how to create and maintain health versus the "disease-care" system that now exists, which has a vested interest in the sick? *The public must be taught how to alter their lifestyle such that disease is not created in the first place—THIS strategy comprises true health care reform.*

Lifestyle is the Answer to the Health Care Crisis

According to Dr. John Knowles, president of the Rockefeller Foundation, "the next major advances in the health of American people will come from the assumption of individual responsibility for one's own health and a necessary change in lifestyle."

And according to the Department of Health, Education and Welfare, "it has become clear that only by preventing disease rather than treating it later, can we hope to achieve any major improvement in the nation's health."

To put these comments into perspective, consider that in the 1990s the major deadly diseases in the U.S. are as follows:

1. ***Cardiovascular diseases*** —directly related to high-fat high-salt intake and insufficient exercise;
2. ***Cancer*** —directly related to high-protein high-fat intake and to smoking;
3. ***Diabetes*** —directly related to high refined-sugar intake and to obesity; and
4. ***Cirrhosis of the liver***— directly related to alcohol and to high refined-sugar intake.

In 1977, the U.S. government, through the Select Senate Committee of Nutrition and Human Needs, issued a revolutionary document entitled "Dietary Goals for the United States," which is the first comprehensive statement ever by any branch of the federal government on risk factors of the American diet. To quote the report:

> "....Our diets have changed radically within the last 50 years with great and very harmful effects on our health. The dietary changes represent as great a threat to public health as smoking. Too much fat, sugar or salt can be and are linked directly to heart disease, cancer, obesity and stroke, among other killer diseases. In all, six of the ten leading causes of death in the U.S. have been linked to diet .....the public wants some guidance, wants to know the truth, and hopefully today we can lay the cornerstone for the building of better health for all Americans through better nutrition."

Specifically, the government's "Dietary Goals for the United States" reads as follows:

1. Increase consumption of fruits, vegetables, and whole grains. Complex carbohydrates should account for 55-60% of caloric intake;
2. Decrease meat consumption, and substitute poultry and fish. Reduce cholesterol consumption to 10% of caloric intake, and balance that with polyunsaturated and monounsaturated fats to about 10% of the caloric intake;

3. Decrease consumption of high-fat foods by 30-40 % of caloric intake. Substitute polyunsaturated fat for saturated fat;
4. Substitute nonfat milk for whole milk;
5. Decrease consumption of butterfat, eggs, and other sources of high cholesterol;
6. Decrease refined sugar consumption by 40%, and foods high in sugar such that they account for about 15% of total caloric intake; and
7. Decrease salt consumption by 50-85%, and foods high in salt content. Reduce salt intake to about three grams a day.

As a result of this report, more and more restaurants and grocery stores have begun catering to vegetarians with low-sugar, low-fat items, and with higher quality and greater variety of produce. *Organic* produce has gained in popularity, and more farmer's markets are now established across the country.

Nevertheless, in the 1990s consider our country's current general lifestyle patterns:

- One of every four Americans uses tobacco;
- Twelve million alcoholics exist in this country;
- Milk is the favorite beverage followed by soda pop, coffee, and tea; the "Basic Four Food Group" plan is still the favored diet, and about 30% eat significantly of pure junk food each day (those high in fat, salt, and/or sugar);
- A growing number of people are eating more fruits and vegetables, and eating less meat, salt, fat, and refined sugar;
- The U.S. has approximately 15 million vegetarians, a trend that is growing as a result of scientific research showing that plant foods combat disease;
- The average life expectancy is about 74 years, which IS NOT due to improved medical care, but is more of a statistical creation because of the drastically reduced

infant and birthing-mother mortality rates that came about as more sanitary conditions have come into practice over the last century and a half.

In the book *Mirage of Health* , Rene Dubos, an eminent bacteriologist and chair holder at the Rockefeller Foundation states that the purported achievements of modern medicine in the decreased incidence of disease, and for increased life expectancy are not all they are cracked-up to be.

Dubos points out that "social reformers" of the early 1800s who campaigned for pure water, better sanitation, and improved living standards were chiefly responsible for decreased mortality rates from so-called infectious disease.

As for life expectancy, Thomas McKenown, in *The Role of Medicine*, explains that statistics purporting to show increased life expectancy rates are misleading since the increase is the consequence of improved living standards and decreased infant mortality. **For those who reach adulthood, life expectancy is barely higher than it was at the turn of the century.**

Health experts are now realizing that crisis medicine has become a bottomless pit. Regardless of how much money is dumped into it, public health is not improved.

Robert Cathcart, chairman of the board of trustees of the American Hospital Association, explains "in the last few years, we have come to recognize that the demand for our services is infinite. We can now begin to act on the lifestyle issue and join others in helping individuals to modify their lifestyle to lead healthier lives, and to reduce the use of expensive services we offer."

From a booklet published by Blue Cross:

"....for the most part, unnoticed bad living habits—not germs, are the big killers in industrialized society. Most Americans choose the way they die. How you live each hour and each day more than anything else will determine what will kill you and when. Over the past 50 years, our unhealthy living habits have grown into a gigantic new disease that kills seven of every ten Americans. The biggest killers today are heart disease, cancer, stroke, cirrhosis of the liver, bronchitis, emphysema and asthma—which kill 76% of the two million people who die each year in this country. There are no vaccines to prevent such threats to life. Cleaning up our lifestyle is the cure. Ironically, rather than improving, lifestyles are getting worse. Changes in diet, smoking, exercise, alcohol consumption and a reduction and a reduction of stress would do more to improve health, than doubling outlays in medical care."

Even though the human body is marvelously designed, it breaks down prematurely. But is this necessary? According to Dr. Lester Breslow, Dean of the School of Public Health at UCLA, "by switching from a bad lifestyle to a healthier one, a person can figure on adding about 14 years to their life."

Scientific and medical professionals are verifying the undeniable fact that our physiology most often prematurely degenerates in those who smoke, drink alcohol, overeat, lead stress-filled lives, eat nutritionally antagonistic "junk foods," lack exercise, get insufficient rest and sleep, and in those who live inharmoniously with others or whose life lacks productive activity.

Insurance consultant Benjamin Lipson says that "bad lifestyles are such a threat to health, that the so-called *average* healthy American with a self-indulgent living pattern, is a far worse insurance risk than a mild adult diabetic who watches their diet."

For all the talk and lip service about disease prevention in this country, it is estimated that less than 5% of the federal government's multi-billion dollar health care budget is directed toward at health promotion and disease prevention.

When the body yields to excessive work, food, drink, and insufficient sleep, instead of thinking about and adjusting the lifestyle to remove illness, people place themselves in the hands of those ***who professionally do their thinking and their care for them.***

No doctor, however, can eat for you, breath for you, sleep for you, or exercise for you. The bottom line is that the individual *must* assume responsibility for his or her own health and *must* be given an accurate education on how to best meet the essentials of health and the genuine needs of the body.

In *Medical Nemesis* , Ivan Illich describes how the medical profession concentrates its resources on treatments for which it gains the largest revenue—rather than on education and prevention of disease which, when effective, would reduce their income and decrease the very need for their services.

Natural Health Care Remedies Used Worldwide

While in this country, the overall approach to health care can be described as "the drugging of America," other countries in Europe and Asia follow a more natural approach that includes natural remedies as recommended by pharmacists and prescribed by doctors.

In Germany, for example, natural substances are used in place of drugs in about 40 illnesses including colds, insomnia, digestive, circulatory and nervous disorders, headaches, high blood pressure, and heart, liver, and kidney diseases—at frequencies ranging from 87% of all prescriptions for colds, to 16% for eye and thyroid problems, and even cancer.

In Western European countries, the 1990 expenditure for alternative therapies was in excess of $1 billion dollars, and in Germany alone, $287 million. From the late 1980s to the early

1990s, the increase in expenditure for these alternative therapies rose 24.2% overall in Europe, 25.5% in Germany, and 35% in the Netherlands over a four year period.

The Government Stifles Our Freedom of Choice in Matters of Health Care

In the U.S., however, the Food and Drug Administration, in the name of "protecting our health," disallows natural remedies from listing medical benefits **even when they are demonstrated in scientific journals.** Instead, the government classifies the natural substance as an unapproved drug, which requires the manufacturer to go through multi-million dollar drug testing that only members of the pharmaceutical cartel can afford.

Special interest groups dominate the health care field in this country. While the FDA removes effective natural remedies in the name of "protecting our health," we can, *without* prescription, buy dangerous over-the-counter drugs, as well as outright poisons, including concentrated sulfuric acid and clorox bleach—but from *natural remedies,* we need "protection" which actually translates into billions of dollars in profits made by the drug companies.

Also, due to the tremendous profit potential, the most dangerous side-effects of drug treatments are often overlooked. While the FDA sees nothing wrong with toxic drugs such as *Prozac* , which is banned or highly restricted in other countries, or with a 51% post-approved risk of new drugs, it needlessly over-regulates manufacturers of natural products in this country.

Instead of embracing alternative health care as it is elsewhere the FDA acts as if it were worthless, and doctors and even patients who use it are not trusted.

Those suffering disease in this country are frequently told by physicians: "Learn to live with it, it's all in your head, it's just hormones, there is nothing that can be done," or "what do you expect at your age?" Patients who question doctors about natural approaches are often told "we are not trained in alternative therapies, they could not possibly be of help."

When patients recover health through natural means and return to the physician for a check-up, they are often greeted with hostility for going outside what Robert Mendelsohn, M.D., calls "the church of modern medicine."

Since alternative medicine in other countries produces healthier individuals and saves money, the FDA is defrauding public health since it makes it difficult to patronize physicians who practice alternative modalities.

Today, the FDA is trying to make amino acid supplements a prescription drug. Previously, tryptophan, for instance, was available for $3.99 per bottle at the local health food store—from a doctor it will cost about $75.00, which includes the fee for the doctor visit and the prescription. This adds about $4 billion-$7 billion to the national health care budget.

The same is true for DHEA (dehydroepinandrosterone). The substance extracted from Mexican yams, is naturally made by our body and is an important "immune stimulant." At UCLA, AIDS patients given DHEA supplements are showing immune system activation. Rather than purchase DHEA at health food stores inexpensively, many costly prescriptions may be written for it, also adding billions to the health care budget.

The FDA is similarly trying to classify vitamins, herbs, amino acids, and co-enzyme Q-10 as drugs (at dosages above a certain level, likely 1.5 times the RDA). **Legislation is now in Congress that will make taking vitamins and supplements possible only with a physician's prescription (Waxman bill HR-3642).**

If this passes, not only will this virtually put health food stores nationwide out of business, thereby closing the only major outlets for organic produce, but the law would also severely limit our health care freedom of choice.

President Clinton himself has said that "dietary supplements like vitamins, minerals, herbs and other nutritional substances have an important role in preventative health...The FDA must not be allowed to infringe on the rights of the millions of Americans who enhance their daily diet with vitamins or other dietary supplements."

The American Dietetic Association has similarly tried in the past, and is still currently attempting to ban and control all nutritional information in the United States. Bills proposed to the House of Representatives by Claude Pepper (HR-6049, HR-6050 and HR-6051) in 1984 and 1985, would have made it illegal for non-credentialed, non-licensed individuals to share health education materials with the public.

The bills died in Congress largely due to public outrage organized by the National Health Federation headquartered in Monrovia, California—an organization devoted to lobbying and to disseminating information that promotes freedom of speech and choice in matters of health care.

Despite these efforts, the ADA continues to pressure government officials to introduce new legislation such as HR-1581 that calls for stiff fines and imprisonment to those in the field of alternative health care who teach other than the status quo.

But the public *must* have the right to choose what works best for them—this country was founded

on such freedom and, without it, our inalienable birthright to healthful living is seriously jeopardized.

The Rockefellers and Carnegies Get Into the Act

And this is not the first time that our access to information on health care has been limited. Have you ever wondered why schools that offer curricula in alternative health-care are NOT accredited? Read the book entitled *Rockefeller Medicine Men: Medicine and Capitalism in America* by E. Richard Brown, published by the University of California Press.

It all started in the early 1900s when the Carnegie and Rockefeller Foundations became heavily involved in funding medical institutions around the country, advocated the philosophy and practice of drug therapy which at the time, was used mostly by the wealthy. (The Rockefellers, by the way, already had a vested interest in selling drugs.)

In 1909, Abraham Flexner was sent by the Carnegie Foundation on a tour of *every* school across the country that offered professional health care training. Flexner decided which schools would be funded with generous grants, based on their willingness to conform to the allopathic model preferred by the Rockefellers and Carnegies.

The *Flexner Report* of 1910 ended health care reform in this country as alternative schools of healing closed—including six of eight black medical schools and *all* that admitted women. **Those who fought closure were vandalized and destroyed.**

Due to their political influence, the Rockefeller and Carnegie Foundations swayed the legislature to pass tough state and federal licensing laws that limited recognition to schools of allopathic medicine, which in effect guaranteed a monopoly on health treatment made available to the public.

Soon, alternative forms of health care were outlawed or driven into the closet, including Homeopathy, midwifery, Natural Hygiene, and very nearly Chiropractic.

Now, with the continuing failures of allopathic medicine, freedom of choice in health care is being re-enlivened and non-medical schools of healing are flourishing, **despite** being non-accredited, as people aggressively search for solutions. Freedom of speech is finally being extended, once again, to the arena of health care due to public demand.

Chapter 4

IS THIS "HEALTH CARE" OR "DISEASE CARE?"

Alfdan Mahler, director of the World Health Organization, says there has been an authoritative mystification of medical care that has led to exploitation of the population by the holders of these mysteries. An unnecessary dependency has been created and the monopolistic position of medicine strengthened.

Currently, the average individual's concept of health and disease is manipulated by economic interests of the medical, drug, and processed food industries via the media. Medical authorities would have us believe that the $800 billion plus health care budget is buying an ever-increasing quality of health in this country. But actually, **current medical practice has very little to do with the promotion of healthful living.**

Our Diseased Society

Despite the medical establishment's portrayal of the United States as a vibrantly healthy populace, the pharmaceutical companies, insurance carriers and other special interest groups have a vested interest in disease. The facts as born out by disease statistics tell a completely different story.

According to the ***Statistical Abstract of the United States 1992*** as published by the U.S. Department of Commerce, and the Bureau of the Census:

- 49% of all Americans suffer AT LEAST one chronic disease;
- One of every five children under age 17 in the U.S. already has developed some chronic disorder;
- Cardiovascular diseases will affect nearly 80% of all Americans and, in 1989, 18.5 million suffered heart conditions;
- In 1990, almost 43% of all deaths in the U.S. were the result of major cardiovascular diseases;
- Cancer will affect 30% of all Americans and 80% of them will die of it;
- In 1991 alone, 1.1 million new cancer cases were diagnosed, and 23% of all deaths were the result of cancer;
- Cancer is the number one cause of death of our children but in many countries almost no cancer exists;
- Arthritic and rheumatic disorders affect 77% of the adult population; currently over 40 million suffer from arthritis;
- In 1990, there were nearly 6.5 million diabetics, and 2% of all deaths were due to diabetes;
- In 1990, 11.6 million suffered from asthma, almost 12 million had bronchitis, and 4% died from pulmonary diseases (asthma, bronchitis, emphysema);
- In 1990, 27.6 million had high blood pressure;

- 16 million Americans suffer ulcers;
- Over 50% in this country suffer chronic digestive disorders;
- 5.4 million suffer frequent indigestion;.
- 4.5 million suffer frequent constipation;
- 11.4 million have hemorrhoids;
- Almost 7 million have urinary infections,
- 50 million are insomniacs who consume over five billion sleeping pills yearly;
- 10 million are migraine sufferers;
- 80 million suffer allergies, and over 21 million hay fever and allergic rhinitis;
- Americans will "come down" with 800 million colds this year; everyday about 90 million aspirins are taken in the U.S. (72 million pounds annually);
- Over 5.8 million suffer from tinnitus or "ringing in the ears";
- 20 million have hearing impairments;
- 7.9 million have visual impairments, and 60% of all Americans have defective vision;
- 5.7 million suffer from cataracts;
- 98.5% of our population have bad teeth, and 31 million have no teeth of their own;
- 70-80% are overweight and 80 million are obese;
- About 10 million Americans suffer psoriasis; another 150 million suffer from acne, eczema, warts and rashes;
- 22 million Americans suffer mental illness;
- Over eight million children are mentally retarded, many caused by drug habits of pregnant mothers;
- Life expectancy for a one-year-old in the U.S. has not increased since the turn of the century;
- Nearly 90% of our children cannot pass a minimum physical fitness test; and
- In 1990, 1.4% of all deaths were due to suicide (nearly 23,000 total).

Regarding destructive lifestyle habits, consider these statistics:

- More than 200 million Americans are hooked on one or more drug habits;
- An estimated 13 billion barbituates and amphetamines are taken annually in the U.S.;
- The worse drug offenders are physicians—they are about 19 times more addicted to narcotics than is the general population;
- Over 100 million Americans drink alcohol, and over 15 million are chronic alcoholics;
- 65% of Americans in 1991 between ages 18-25 were current users of alcohol; over 25% from age 12-17; and 55% of those over 26 years of age;
- About 60 million use tobacco, and over 600 billion cigarettes are smoked annually in this country;
- In 1988, almost 168 million people 20 years and older smoked cigarettes in the U.S.;
- In 1991, nearly 12% of 12-17 year olds were smokers; over 35% of those between ages 18-25; and nearly 30% age 26 and above;
- Americans consume 250 billion cups of coffee regularly; and
- The average American eats over 125 pounds of sugar each year, and 95% of our population are sugar addicts.

Finally, the U.S. Public Health Service recognizes:

- Approximately 3.5 million of us as being healthy —**only 1.5%** of our population;
- About one billion annual visits are made to physicians in our country;
- 40 million Americans spend time in the hospital each year;
- Another quarter of a billion visit hospital emergency rooms and clinics;

- In 1990, over 11.6 million out-patient surgeries were performed in the U.S., a 265% increase over 1980 figures;
- In 1989, over 23 million in-patient surgeries were performed;
- Currently, about 25 million surgeries are performed yearly; and finally
- Five million of us each year are seriously poisoned by physician's drugs and require hospitalization as a result of iatrogenic (physician generated) disease.

The U.S. is actually among the most diseased industrialized nations in the world—in spite of the fact that we spend the most on health care, have the most physicians, the most surgeons, hospitals, nurses, and nursing homes than anywhere else worldwide.

The Solution—
Don't Get Sick In the First Place

In order to preserve health, the causes of disease must be avoided, which implies living according to our natural mandate.

In other words, we need to learn to live healthfully to begin with so as NOT to bring on costly disease. More importantly, we need to understand the nature of disease and how to best fulfill our physiological requisites so that we aid healing when sickness occurs, rather than further complicating the disease process.

The quality of human health should not depend on who can turn the largest profit. Our health care system is driven by profits, not by educating the public on how to maintain and preserve their well-being.

And THIS is the purpose of this book—to shed

light on our actual biological requirements in maintaining health and to describe the true nature of disease.

The public has come to expect a great deal from contemporary health care, perhaps too much. **Due to rising costs, the only rational choice left is for each individual to regain control over his or her own health by learning and then consistently meeting his or her physiological needs and the essentials of health.**

We have to take charge of our own health by returning to the basics: nutrition, biologically correct health practices, and by avoiding manufactured chemicals in our food and environment.

Nutrition Education "Inadequate" in U.S. Medical Schools

Historically, nutrition has played a peripheral role in medical treatment. Recently, however, many doctors are recognizing that this omission is a major oversight. Moreover, medical practitioners must be aware that good nutrition is not an "alternative therapy"—rather, it is a fundamental component of the essentials of health and the biological needs of life.

The lack of nutritional education in almost all Western medical schools, combined with a lack of funding, has prevented serious attention from being focused on this aspect of health maintenance and disease prevention.

Since nutrients cannot be patented, pharmaceutical companies have little profit motive to fund such research. Even though tens of thousands of published articles confirm the influence of nutrition on disease prevention, many doctors have largely ignored its central role in patient care.

Back in 1985, just after the National Research Council released a report on the quality of training provided at medical schools throughout the United States, *Tufts University Diet & Nutrition Letter* wrote the following: **"Inadequate describes the nutrition education that most physicians receive while studying to become doctors."**

In the 1990s, this has not changed, according to the results of a new nationwide survey of nutrition-related practices of physicians—and that's despite ever increasing knowledge of the links between dietary habits and the risks of major killer diseases including cancer and heart disease.

Survey coordinator Barbara Levine, Ph.D, director of the Nutrition Information Center at New York Hospital-Cornell Medical Center in New York, points out that of the 30,000 surveys mailed out to physicians, only 11% responded. The 27,000 doctors who ignored the survey probably are even *less* interested in incorporating the science of nutrition into their practice.

What we need to do, says Dr. Levine, is to develop ways to encourage physicians to make nutrition a standard part of patient care. In medical school, doctors should be required to apply nutrition to their *own* lives as well as to their patients. In addition, Dr. Levine suggests that competence in nutrition should be demonstrated before licensure to practice medicine is granted.

True Health Reform is *Self-Health Care*— An Introduction to Natural Hygiene

The public wants guidance in SELF-health care—how to live and adjust their lifestyle such that the causes of disease are avoided. The public needs straightforward knowledge of how their physiology operates and how to best meet the essentials of health.

Health is the preeminent desire of our age. A precise and practical knowledge of the conditions of health and of the circumstances which induce disease—as well as the methods of removing disease WITHOUT generating future iatrogenic disease, (illness that is, *caused* by prescription drugs and medical intervention) is a great need of our time.

Fortunately, there does exist a healing art that is very efficient in removing disease and in restoring the body to a condition of health.

This healing art is distinguished in both theory and practice from medical science, from chiropractic, osteopathy, homeopathy, herbology, ayurveda, acupuncture, and all other systems of healing—**for it is concerned SOLELY with removing the cause of disease, whereas others are content to treat the end-points (symptoms) of pathology.** In this sense, it belongs in a class by itself as it is diametrically opposed to all other healing modalities.

Almost as old as our country, is a ***Self*** **Health-Care System** that is still in operation today. Early in the 19th century, ***Natural Hygiene*** was initially formalized after **NATURE** upon which it is based, and after **HYGIENE**—the science of health.

The Hygienic Health-Care System was originally developed in the United States by Isaac Jennings, M.D., of Fairfield, Connecticut, and was slowly elaborated in both its philosophical and theoretical aspects and in its practical applications by Russell Thatcher Trall, M.D., and Sylvester Graham in the early 1800s.

In the 1850s and 1860s, Dr. Trall did much original research that further developed Hygiene. After their deaths, others continued the Hygienic System in this country by establishing a number of sanitaria and organizations throughout America that *still* carry out hygienic methods in the regeneration of health and that disseminate educational programs to the public (see appendix A for listings.)

With the coming of both the Civil War and Pasteur's "germ theory" hygienic health reform in the 1800s declined. Modern medicine found a powerful ally in the drug trade, and this alliance created a monopoly on almost all avenues of health information and learning.

Though it never died, Natural Hygiene continued to decline despite such champions as Bernard McFadden, James C. Jackson, M.D., Robert Walter, M.D., Felix Oswald and others. In the 1920s, Dr. Herbert M. Shelton arrived on the scene as a giant in reviving Hygienic Health Care. (A brief but more detailed sketch of the history of Natural Hygiene is outlined in appendix B).

The title ***"Natural Hygiene"*** distinguishes the employment of influences and substances that have a constitutional relation to the living organism from the employment of those that are abnormal, anti-vital, and which have no normal relation to life.

The term ***"Natural"*** means those processes that are unhampered by artificial, or man-made forces. As used here, it also means that to which we are biologically adapted—the sum total of our heritage from nature.

The word ***"Hygiene"*** is derived from ***"Hygeia"***—the Greek goddess of health and, as used throughout Natural Hygiene literature, means the science of health, pertaining to everything that bears upon human welfare.

The Greek words ***"hygies"*** and ***"hygiene"*** are derived from the Sanskrit root *"ugras"* which means vigorous. Also from this root comes the word *"vegetable."* The Latin *"vegetus"* similarly means vigorous, active, and lively. ***"Hygiene"*** is defined as the science and art of maintaining community and individual health, and **"hygienics"** are the principles and methods of preserving or promoting well-being.

Natural Hygiene, then, is the branch of biology that investigates the conditions upon which health depends, the means by which it may be sustained, and the natural methodologies whereby health is restored when it has been lost or impaired.

It is concerned with those principles applicable to human life, the study of the primordial requisites of health and the application of these basic essentials toward consistently meeting life's needs. Natural Hygiene studies *total* human nutrition and well-being (meaning the sum of ALL body processes) **and involves the practical application of these guiding principles in daily living.**

Hygienic Health-Care has long stated that the essentials of health include:

- A plant-based diet which emphasizes fresh raw fruits and vegetables;
- The importance of environment including pure air, pure water, healthy working conditions, and aesthetic beauty;
- Appropriate activity, including balanced exercise, rest, work, and play; and
- A sound psychology predicated on self-responsibility self-acceptance, self-awareness, and self-mastery.

Specifically, Natural Hygiene involves the study of the following relationships:

1. How our specific lifestyle choices relate to health and disease;
2. How health and disease relate to the functional WHOLENESS of the human system;
3. The relationship between the human body and the environment; and
4. The relationship between the mind and body.

Hygienic Health Care is based on a fundamental understanding of how the body operates—and how human needs and physiological capacities and limitations are all interrelated.

Natural Hygiene is easy to understand. Its message is simple and not concealed by incomprehensible scientific jargon or by the technical nomenclature of modern medicine.

Hygienic Self-Health Care has no "magic bullets" to sell, no wonder drugs, herbs or panaceas that promise to create well-being. Instead, Hygiene points to our biological adaptations and the underlying laws of physiology that provide guidance in attaining and preserving health—and this is why it works.

The Hygienic system of the 19th century was obviously not as efficient as that of today. Although it had the same basic premises, its practical application had yet to be perfected. In fact, it can *still* be improved even though most objectives of Natural Hygiene are now easily attainable since splendid health in both youth and old age is now possible as long as we choose to live accordingly. In this sense, Hygienic Health Care has scored a major victory.

And once more, why does Natural Hygiene work? Because it *fully* cooperates with the underlying principles that govern our ***Self***-healing body. To understand the significance of this, we need to take a brief, yet closer look at our truly remarkable physiology.

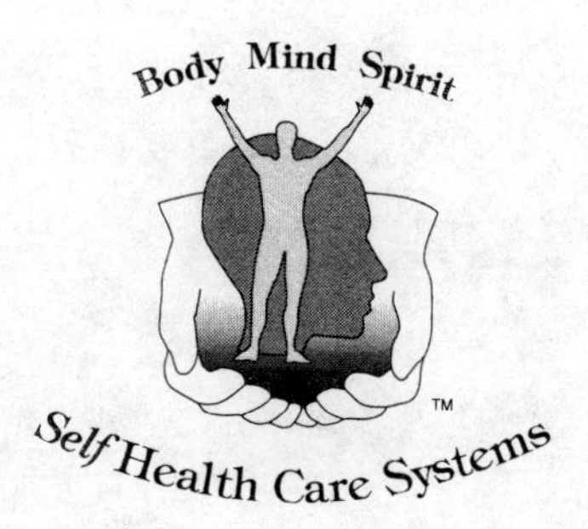
Body Mind Spirit
Self Health Care Systems
TM

<u>SECTION II</u>

THE SOLUTION:

HEALTH REFORM BASED ON OUR BIOLOGICAL ADAPTATIONS

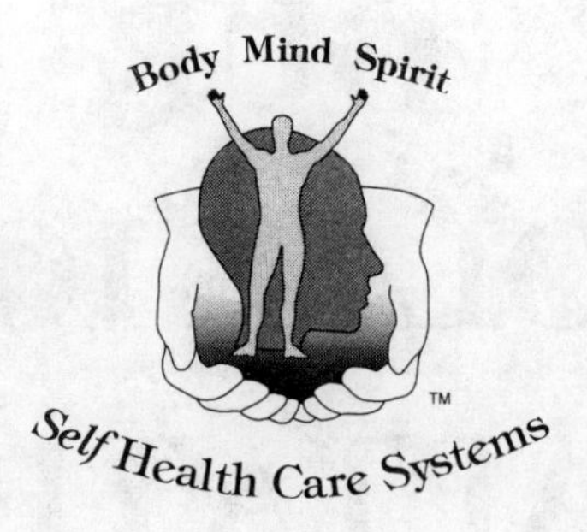
Body Mind Spirit
Self Health Care Systems

Chapter 5

THE INCREDIBLE ORGANIZING POWER OF THE HUMAN BODY—PHENOMENAL FACTS OF PHYSIOLOGY

The mature human body is a universe of some 100 trillion cells—highly complex units of life that collectively live in harmony under normal circumstances, which include those healthy conditions that ideally meet the body's needs within the context of its biological character.

The human body has developed over eons of time and has perfected itself over millions of years, through countless thousands of generations within certain narrowly defined adaptational parameters.

Like the seasons of nature, the vital actions of the body express themselves in rhythms and cycles. These actions are subject to the direction of the body's immense intelligence that adapts the raw materials of the environment for our use and continued survival.

Through the force of our nervous system the body's wisdom maintains the matter of our physical structure in a completely cooperative cellular society which organizes over 400 trillion parts and literally billions of nerve cell galaxies to control the pumping of blood, the breathing of air, and the sweating that occurs through literally miles of skin cells.

From the moment of conception, our body has developed from a single microscopic ovum into its present state of approximately 75-100 trillion cells. The human body has more moving parts and is considerably more complicated than any man-made machine ever constructed.

There are more than 600 muscles and 200 bones in the body, all of which counter-balance each other to maintain posture, alignment and coordinated body form. Unlike machines, the human body is a living, growing entity which through proper care is subject to positive constructive change.

The body loses and replaces from 300 billion-800 billion cells each day (some ten million each second)—mostly red corpuscles from the bloodstream. The average person loses about 70 billion cells each day from the digestive tract alone, as well as losing the entire lining of the mouth. The total amount of cells lost daily depends primarily upon how destructive the lifestyle practices of the individual are.

The body also contains about 25 trillion blood cells, whose average life expectancy is only around 30 days or so. To replace these is a constant process—as you read this sentence, your body has created seven to ten million new blood cells each second through the process called *mitosis.*

Simultaneously, deceased cells decompose and are recycled by white corpuscles. If body vitality, white blood cell capacity, and our eliminative organs are not equal to the task of recycling and removing these body wastes, they become a serious problem and a source of disease.

Incredibly, the circulatory system itself is composed of 60,000-70,000 miles of blood and lymphatic vessels tightly packed (mostly in the form of minute capillaries) which circulate about five to six quarts of blood.

To accomplish this, the heart beats about 2.5 billion times in an average lifetime, driving the blood supply each moment to every cell in the body in order to cleanse and nourish the entire system—that's well over 10,000 quarts of blood pumped through the circulatory system EACH DAY, and 220 million quarts over a lifetime.

To achieve this feat, a normal heart beats over 103,000 times DAILY or pulsates about 40 million times each year. In fifty years, it contracts and expands about two billion times. Think of the enormous amount of vital energy required to carry on just this work alone.

If we live by meeting our biological needs regularly, while making a conscious effort to avoid toxic substances and influences, our heart will pump some three billion times over 100 years if given the chance. But the greatest enemies to normal heart function are perverted nutrition and a lethargic lifestyle.

Likewise with the brain. It is estimated we lose about 100,000 brain cells per day through normal attrition—never to be replaced. A single bout with alcohol however, is estimated to increase the days loss to over a million cells.

Even those who are healthy lose about 1 billion neurons throughout their lifetime at an average of about 18 million per year. This loss is compensated for by the remaining nerve cell's branchlike-filaments called *dendrites*, which connect neurons into functional networks.

The brain itself is composed of about 50 billion neurons, each involved in transmitting messages throughout the body. Scientists say that nerve cells do not reproduce—once they die, neurons are not replaced.

Even the healthiest of us lose approximately 100,000 brain cells daily. But even at this rate, it would take 150 years to lose 10% of our brain capacity. Unfortunately, we often squander this precious organ and become senile in our sixties, seventies or eighties with perhaps 50% loss of cerebral matter due to destructive lifestyle practices.

And don't forget about our oxygen needs. Daily, the lungs draw in about 20,000 breaths of inhaled air during which time the average adult inhales about 777,000 cubic inches of air.

During this day's work, the equivalent of 125 barrels of blood are purged of carbon dioxide and other toxic gases, and then re-oxygenated. A pair of normal lungs contains approximately a billion tiny air cells. If spread out on a flat surface, the cells would cover an area some 40 x 50 feet.

Finally, the "wrapping paper" is pretty incredible too! It is estimated that every square inch of the skin is made up of 19.5 billion individual cells. The skin contains about seven million pores, representing some seven miles of "sewer-lines" which serve as exit passages for wastes both generated by and introduced into the system.

All of this incredibly complex activity and organization of the body is orchestrated automatically, without requiring the attention of our conscious awareness.

These facts and figures are presented so that you can realize that **the incredible programming and unknowable powers that developed the body are all that is needed for its non-ceasing, self-perpetual maintenance and repair.**

The Body's Innate Intelligence

The body is the best arbiter of its needs—it is autonomous, and operates from a cumulative fount of wisdom spawned by countless centuries of evolution that our conscious intellect can never hope to emulate.

The body's inherent intelligence is illustrated by its actions during growth, healing, digestion, autolysis, fasting, and protein formation (among numerous others).

For example, there are over 100,000 different proteins created by the body from recycled and ingested protein molecules which are first broken down into component amino acids and then re-synthesized by the system. It is said that the body renews itself some 160 times in 70 years, but this statement is a bit misleading since the constant renewal process is continuous until death.

The body's complex wisdom is apparent in even the simple act of eating an apple. At least 191 known chemical compounds are contained in a plain apple each of which plays an important role in human nutrition. When eaten, over 1,300 chemical reactions occur to break the apple down into its component molecules which are then dispatched to EXACTLY the areas of the body where they are required. Pectin goes to the large intestine; vitamin C to the skin; vitamin A to the eye's retina; and so on 191 times.

Of the 160,000 edible plants on this earth, our digestive system can convert these into brain, bone, heart, muscles, and energy to keep us alive. The body alone knows what it needs—don't think those industries who manufacture instant breakfasts, imitation orange juice, bleached white bread, vitamin pills, and nutritional supplements have the slightest idea what the body requires.

Our wonderfully developed intellect is humbled by and

can never improve on the wisdom that brought us here, and which allows us to survive from day to day.

There is NO exact way of consciously determining the *precise* needs of the body—no human mind can possibly prescribe human-formulated doses and materials to meet our constantly changing systemic needs. Only our body's inborn intelligence can do that, and once we consciously begin our transition into healthier living without outside interference, the body starts to balance itself and regains homeostasis.

Body wisdom cannot be pinpointed anywhere in particular within the body, for intelligence resides as a guiding feature in every cell, tissue and, indeed, within the very fabric of our existence.

Each cell possesses more knowledge and expertise (embodied within DNA) than the whole human race collectively on the conscious level. We know intelligence is there when we perceive how extensive it is but, by and large, our population is unaware of their own bodies' tremendous faculties.

The wisdom and "know-how" lying behind the body's functioning is immense. Maintaining delicate blood acid/alkaline balance, glucose levels, body temperature and blood pressure requires tremendously complicated physiological mechanisms. The body's ability to maintain its steady state, called *homeostasis,* requires far more complicated systems than the finest computer engineer could design.

(Homeostasis refers to the vital balance in the body with respect to various physiological functions such as body temperature, heart rate, blood pressure, blood sugar, water content, etc., and to the proper chemical compositions of fluids and tissues).

The body has highly intricate control and regulatory mechanisms that maintain an ideal body equilibrium in all except overwhelmingly adverse circumstances.

Innate genetic intelligence (under the guidance of the brain and nervous system) operates the body's metabolic processes and its trillions of cells. This intelligence is inherent and automatic. The logistics involved in nourishing every single one of the 100 trillion body cells and their internal population of quadrillions of mitochondria requires intelligence well beyond our intellectual command.

The body is constantly at work maintaining homeostasis and the most ideal operating conditions possible. It is only after repeated, constant abuse that the healing forces fail as they become overwhelmed and exhausted. Normality is re-established as the conditions of health are restored to the general lifestyle.

As mentioned previously, the human body has more moving parts and is considerably more complicated than any man-made machine.

Outside of the human body, man cannot create a single drop of blood, cannot produce a single living cell, cannot mend a broken bone, and cannot repair a simple wound. All he may do is remove all interfering factors, whether internal or external, and supply the normal conditions for life. After that, our organs and life processes automatically do the work of maintenance and healing.

We must respect our body intelligence—it is far greater than ALL the accumulated recorded knowledge of the human race, ***for the same forces which guided the development of the single celled, fertilized ovum into the highly complex 100 trillion celled living organism, continues today to oversee the welfare of the body.*** The body is the master of its domain. Place full confidence in the powers of the body.

The very structure and function of the body—its physiological capabilities and limitations—dictate certain unchanging principles which determine how and in what manner the human organism needs to be nourished to remain in superb health.

General law and orderliness underlies life (as described by biology and physiology), which, if defied in our eating and lifestyle, does not allow for our health to be maintained.

Our biological adaptations therefore—the way our body developed through evolution while in a pristine state of nature—determine our needs and how we should meet them. So long as we respect the body's integrity by consistently meeting its needs, our system is its own master.

Our physiology is programmed from the moment of conception to develop from a microscopic, singled-celled ovum into a superbly functioning, intelligent human being—and to automatically carrying on the innumerable metabolic functions of life while keeping us well and happy until a natural death occurs at a much advanced age.

As such, we may place absolute and full reliance upon the intelligence underlying our system, so long as we provide it with life's essentials.

As we no longer live in a natural environment, we must learn and educate ourselves as to how to balance our diet and lifestyle (since this is no longer instinctive as it is throughout the animal kingdom). Knowledge of food and correct lifestyle habits is essential if we are to maintain health and vigor.

We can consciously choose to respect and supply our bodily, mental, emotional, and spiritual needs or we can intentionally (or unintentionally) ignore them and suffer the consequences.

The Importance of Body Cleanliness and Purity of Our Body Fluids

There are two aspects to keeping the body pure: **internal cleanliness;** and **external cleanliness.** By far, the most important of these is maintaining internal purity, for if the normal biological processes responsible for maintaining internal cleanliness ceased, we would literally die within minutes from the poisons of our metabolic wastes. Only the functioning of the body's "drainage system" prevents metabolic by-products from quickly extinguishing life.

External cleanliness and a sweet smelling body actually depend upon a clean interior. No amount of soap and deodorants will erase the foul effects of morbid material constantly being excreted through the skin—we must first, purify our interior.

Most action of body cleanliness on the outside amounts to cleaning the exterior of a garbage can while paying little or no attention to the can's contents. EXTERNAL CLEANSING IS A MECHANICAL AND NOT A CHEMICAL PROCESS.

The human body contains hundreds of defensive mechanisms (mostly in the form of white blood cells) to protect and continuously purify itself against the ravages of poisons.

White blood cells are the body's first line of defense against foreign materials that circulate within the bloodstream. They are our sanitation engineers maintaining the purity of the tissues, lymph, and body fluids. If poisons, bacteria, fungi (yeast), metabolic wastes, cooked food debris, or other foreign substances enter the blood, they are engulfed by our white blood cells.

White blood cells tolerate nothing that should not be in the blood. Some of what is apprehended is recycled as food, especially body wastes and organic materials, including alien blood introduced via transfusion.

In the aftermath of eating cooked food or taking drugs, for instance, our white blood cell count is likely to rise to between 12,000-20,000 per cubic millimeter of blood in a phenomenon called *leucocytosis*. White cells, including lymphocytes, plasma cells, monocytes, basophils, neutrophils, eosinophils, and granulocytes clear the circulation of toxic materials.

After clearing the bloodstream of toxic debris or poisons, our white blood cell count decreases back to "normal," about 4,300-7,000 per cubic millimeter of blood.

This pathological norm is based on the general populace who routinely consume junk food, cooked foods, condiments, soft drinks, teas, coffee, tobacco, and fermented foods, all of which cause abnormal proliferation of white blood cells.

On the other hand, those who consume a purer, clean-burning diet of predominantly raw fruits, vegetables, nuts and seeds have white cell counts well below 4,300—*and are regarded as immunodeficient!!*

The truth is, of course, that those who are REALLY suffering from immunodeficiency diseases have destroyed their bodies' capacity to generate white blood cells from constantly ingesting drugs or massive transfusions, whereas the healthy body is parsimonious—it harvests its resources strictly according to need.

The body is very stingy in that it does not maintain faculties beyond what it requires. Healthy individuals, for instance, whose bloodstreams are pure, have lower white blood cell counts, holding the remainder in reserve within bone marrow, capillaries, and lymph nodes for times of emergency.

The body's tremendous capacity to throw-off toxins is drained away by our poor lifestyle, however. The average American poisons him or herself some 20-40 times DAILY (to be discussed at more length in upcoming chapters), and each bout lowers body vitality until chronic disease cripples us.

Our physiology takes enormous punishment via our modern lifestyle and yet survives. Over 50% of Americans suffer some serious chronic illness. Forty-five percent of Americans die of heart disease; another 20% from cancer; Americans suffer some 800 million colds a year; and over 50% of all meals eaten in this country end up causing indigestion. Even though some 75% of our population lives to age 70-80, we are rarely healthy.

If we are to escape the degenerative diseases that ravage our majority, we must learn to recognize what the body needs and what to avoid. Otherwise, gradually, erosion of health occurs, according to the individuals inherited constitution, and the extensiveness of the biological and physiological infractions.

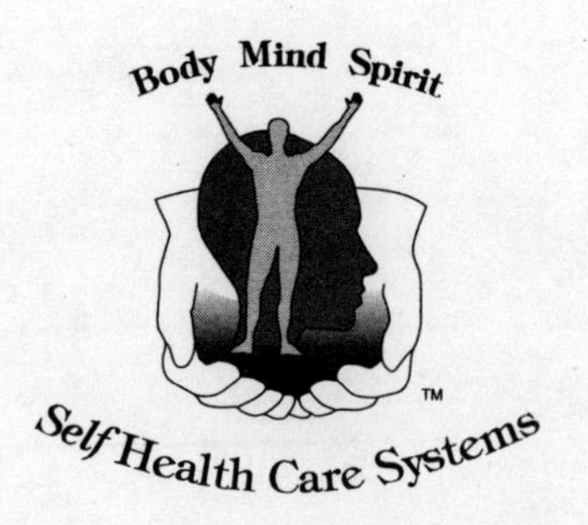
Body Mind Spirit
Self Health Care Systems

Chapter 6

DIET MUST BE ADAPTED TO OUR BIOLOGY— DETERMINING OUR NATURAL DIETARY NEEDS

The highest powers of the body are maintained only if the elements on which the body optimally thrives are continuously supplied to it. Just as an automobile runs best on the finest gasoline for which it was designed and becomes sluggish and grinds to a halt on kerosene, so too the body will operate at its highest level on the finest foods and influences to which, in its millions of years of development, it has become biologically adapted.

In other words, the body works most efficiently when our diet consists of those foods to which we are biologically designed to eat since *these* foods contain no major toxins or impediments that hamper normal function and repair. And what does this ideal diet consist of and how are we certain of its accuracy? As always, **we turn to nature for answers.**

The Role of Biological Adaptations

Every living creature exists with specific qualities, attributes, potentials, and limitations inherent to the organism which define its nature. There are certain clearly delineated characteristics in the anatomy and physiology of various species which invariably center around their natural diet—and in fact, the diet of most animals is defined by their inherent food-gathering equipment.

Biological adaptations describe the faculties an organism or species has developed to meet its requirements in the environment in which it lives. What is *"natural"* to a particular species depends upon its environmental adaptations—to what it has become accustomed to while living in a pristine state of nature. And conversely, that which is *contrary* to an organism's biological heritage is abnormal and unnatural to it.

Every animal has a class of food to which it is naturally adapted. *Herbivores* (cattle, rabbits, elephants, horses, sheep, etc.) are equipped to handle an exclusive leaf/grass diet. *Graminivores* (primarily birds) thrive on the grains of various grasses. *Carnivores* (dogs, cats, lions, tigers, wolves, etc.) eat meat, but even they cannot thrive on an all-meat diet. *Frugivores* (apes, gorillas, chimpanzees, monkeys, orangutans etc.) thrive primarily on fruits.

Those foods and influences to which animals are biologically adapted are those deemed "natural" to its disposition as derived by the sum total of their biological heritage from millions of years of evolution. Cumulative adaptations in each species over eons of time determines their natural dietary needs.

Biology studies organisms in their native environment to which they have been accustomed for hundreds of thousands of years. Different organisms have developed their own characteristics which allow them to live and prosper.

The koala bear of Australia, for instance, is adapted to eating a variety of gum leaves. The giraffe's long neck allows it to feed on the foliage of trees. The lion's fangs and claws allow it to kill and render animals for food. The eagle's keen eyesight and powerful claws make it a formidable predator of ground rodents and small game. Carnivores have become adapted to eating other animals. Non-carnivorous animals have adapted to eating vegetable matter as food.

Dietary adaptations more than anything else determine the features and characteristics of all creatures. ***HUMANS ARE NOT AN EXCEPTION.*** It is a basic premise of Natural Hygiene that man (like other creatures in the animal kingdom) was provided by nature with all the materials and conditions required to maintain health and strength.

Animals in nature intuitively restrict themselves to a limited variety of foods to which they are specifically adapted. **We must conclude that man also is intended to partake only of those foods to which HE is physiologically adapted in order to live healthfully.**

Man should be studied as a member of the whole biological community, and compared anatomically and physiologically with other animals to ascertain his true natural dietary requirements.

When considering the character of human anatomy and physiology relative to our natural diet we must do so within the context of nature, rather than in the artificial environment of modern life. In this way, we consider our natural foods as those that are consonant with our physiological faculties, rather than those that we have "acquired a taste for."

Tradition and popularity are the poorest ways to determine a proper diet. **The *only* authority you should rely on when it comes to determining what foods are best to eat is *your own body.*** It is the anatomy and physiology of your own body that makes foods "acceptable" or "harmful" in the diet.

Determining our natural diet is not a matter of belief—for its basis lies in scientific fact regarding our biological, biochemical, anatomical, and physiological features.

Our biological adaptations have been spurred on by stress over eons of time, and by the need to adapt. Biological adaptations are slow, requiring extremely long periods of time to evolve. If there is a failure to adapt or if environmental change is too rapid, the danger of extinction exists. Distress consists of situations and events with which we cannot cope or which impose great difficulty. Continuous distress speedily exhausts the organism and contributes to its premature demise.

Recent changes in our *external* environment do not alter our biological adaptations, our internal makeup, nor our natural needs in order to establish optimum well-being. Our highly industrialized environment involves more *social* adaptations or accommodations, and not physical or anatomical changes. By living according to our natural adaptations we can actually withstand the stress of modern life far better than if we transgress our biological mandate and our natural needs.

The first question in forming a scientific, rather than commercial approach, to human nutrition is this: of what biological disposition is the human organism? What is our natural food? Are we true graminivores and herbivores (vegetarians) who thrive on lettuce, grasses, raw grains, celery, etc., as do horses, cows and sheep?

Are we true carnivores who secure their nutrient needs

not only from flesh, but also from blood, bones, gristle, and offal from the fresh kill? Are we frugivores who can thrive on a diet of bananas, grapes, apples, oranges, or melons meal after meal? Or are we natural omnivores who thrive in health regardless of the foodstuffs consumed?

Man's digestive system and physiology determines his optimum diet. By understanding the physiological processes that accompany food digestion and absorption, proper dietary habits can be scientifically determined.

The major physical processes of digestion are basically the same for all human beings regardless of race. These processes should be studied in relation to human health in order to develop an accurate science of our true nutritional and dietary needs.

A wealth of information exists about the physiology of food digestion and absorption. Unfortunately, however, **"modern" nutritional science has often depended upon experiments on rats and artificially induced deficiencies in erroneous attempts to determine our dietary needs.**

A more reasonable approach to ascertain our actual dietary nature is to study human anatomy and physiology. In this way, characteristics of our proper diet can be deduced that are in accordance with the inherent nature and anatomical makeup of mankind.

This approach does not depend on contrived animal experiments, nor is it biased by commercial processed-food interests (including the meat and dairy industries) who have dictated for decades our traditional diet.

Profit is not the motive of this investigation—health is. Human physiological capabilities and predispositions are the proper basis in determining our actual dietary needs.

Today's "nutritionists" are subservient to the "basic four

food groups" concept as perpetuated by big industry in this country. According to these nutritionists, humans do not have a fixed diet as other animals in nature—rather, we are omnivorous creatures that are supposed to partake of numerous foods at virtually every meal in order to satisfy our nutritional requirements.

The Human Body is Different From That of Other Species

Anatomically, however, humans are most **un**like herbivores, carnivores, and omnivores in most physical features. Every organ and system differs radically because each is suited to the animals respective mode of food acquisition and digestion.

When we examine other species, the anatomical features of humans are very dissimilar from carnivores (dogs, cats, eagles, etc.); from omnivores (hogs, pigs, bears, etc.); from herbivores (horses, cattle, sheep, etc.); and from insectivores. Humans are unique in the animal kingdom but are remarkably similar both physiologically and in temperament to apes and primates who are frugivores.

Science Verifies That Humans Are Frugivores

Recent research by anthropologists shows that we had an arboreal past—our ancestors were once tree dwellers. At that time, we depended upon products of the tree, and later upon the fruits of stalk and vine for our sustenance.

Dr. Alan Walker, an anthropologist of John Hopkins University in Maryland, has done research showing that humans were once *exclusively* fruit eaters.

By careful examination of fossil teeth and fossilized human remains with electron microscopes and other sophisticated tools, Dr. Walker and his colleagues are absolutely certain that our ancestors, until relatively recently, were total fruitarians. These findings were reported in depth in the May 15, 1979 issue of the *New York Times* .

The essence of Walker's research is that even though humans have adopted omnivorous eating practices, our anatomy and physiology have not changed—we remain biologically a species of fruit eaters.

The human digestive system has been adapted to a diet of fruits and vegetables for more than 60 million years of development. A few thousand years of perverted eating will not change our dietary requirements for optimum health.

The position that humans occupy in the animal kingdom is that of the *Primate order*, which means that, from the point of view of anatomy, our closest animal relatives are the anthropoid apes (anthropoid means "resembling man" or "man-like"). This group of animals include gorillas, monkeys, chimps, etc., all of whom are classified as frugivores, meaning fruit eaters.

From the perspective of physiology, man's biology and digestive apparatus most closely resemble his closest cousin in the animal kingdom—the orangutan. Humans developed on fruits just as our simian and other primitive relatives in nature. In consequence, some anthropologists and biologists have classified humans as frugivores.

Specifically, the biological, biochemical, anatomical, and physiological features of man place him in the class of frugivores as indicated by our dental formula and structure of our teeth, the length and structure of our digestive system, the relative size of our liver and kidneys, the biochemistry of our saliva and other digestive secretions, the function of our skin, the number and position of the mammary glands, the position of our eyes, the function of our sweat pores, the character of our hands and nails, the position of our reproductive organs, the character of the human placenta, and our method of physical transportation—all these factors indicate our constitutional nature and biological heritage as a frugivore.

Oddly, many anthropologists classify man as an omnivore, meaning an "everything eater" like pigs, hogs, and the scavengers. Man indeed does eat everything. But if we compare the human anatomy and digestive system to the primates who are natural frugivores, we find they are virtually identical.

The intestines are both 12 times the length of the body trunk; the large intestine (colon) is convoluted, slowing the passage of food; the teeth of both man and the primates are the same; saliva is alkaline; and our skin has pores to aid in the elimination of wastes. Herbivores (deer, cows, horses, etc.) are similar but not identical. Their intestines are generally 10 times the length of their trunk.

These scientific facts raise the emotionally charged, perennial question: are we biologically a race of plant-eaters (herbivores/vegetarians), or are we true masticators of flesh (carnivores/meat-eaters)? Let's examine the scientifc facts.

Chapter 7

ARE WE NATURAL MEAT-EATERS, OR ARE WE NATURAL VEGETARIANS?

Most "nutritionists" even assert that we have definite carnivorous leanings, and some have even termed our incisor teeth "fangs" in defense of their erroneous position that humans are natural meat-eaters!! If you look at the various species in the animal kingdom, each is equipped with teeth that are ideally suited to masticate a particular type of food.

Herbivores (like the cow) have 24 molars, eight jagged incisors in the lower jaw and a horny palate in the upper jaw. The jaws move vertically, laterally, forward, and backward, enabling the herbivore to tear and grind coarse grasses. The omnivore (like the hog) has tusk-like canines allowing them to dig up roots.

Frugivores (like the gorilla) have 32 teeth—sixteen in each jaw including four incisors, two cuspids, four bicuspids, and six molars. The cuspids are adapted for cracking nuts, and the uniform articulation of the teeth enables the frugivore to mash and grind fruits.

On the contrary, carnivores (like the cat family) have markedly developed canines that are long, sharp, cylindrical, pointed, and set apart from the other teeth. Fangs and sharp pointed teeth that penetrate and kill, that rip and tear flesh are a feature of all true carnivores (except certain birds). The powerful jaws of the carnivore move only vertically, and are ideal for ripping and tearing flesh which is swallowed virtually whole and then acted upon by extremely potent gastric juices.

Man's teeth are not designed for tearing flesh as in the wolf or dog, but rather compare closely with other fruit-eating animals. Man's teeth correspond almost identically to the gorilla's and other frugivores. The complete absence of spaces between human teeth characterizes him as the archetype frugivore.

The "canine" teeth of man are short, stout, and slightly triangular. They are less pronounced and developed than the gorilla's, who rarely (if ever) indulges in flesh in its natural state. To term our incisor teeth "fangs" or even to liken them as such, is outrageous.

Man's canines in no way resemble the long, round, slender canines of the true carnivore. Man's teeth are not curved or sharp like the wolve's or tiger's, nor are they wide and flat like the grass and grain-eating species. Man's teeth are actually like the fruit-eating monkey's, and man's mouth is best suited for eating succulent fruits and vegetables. It would be extremely difficult, if not impossible, for man to eat *raw* flesh without the aid of fork and knife.

Natural carnivores have the inherent anatomical equipment provided as their birthright with which to apprehend, capture, kill, and rend their quarry. Dogs have powerful jaws that inflict fatal wounds to their prey.

Humans, however, have no sharp claws for tearing; no sharply pointed fangs for slashing; nor are our eyes or olfactory senses well developed for hunting—and neither is our body designed to run fast enough to capture prey.

Humans cannot grab animals in their mouth as do dogs, coyotes, wolves, jackals, lions, tigers, or cats—we instead inflict more damage with our hands and brute strength. Humans do, however, have marvelous fingers, thumbs, and limbs for reaching, climbing and grabbing. Our natural food gathering capacity is very similar to the chimpanzee's.

Fruitarians of the primate order also have revolving joints in their shoulder, wrist, and elbow joints which allow for free movement in all directions. Frugivores have soft pliable, sensitive hands and fingers with opposable thumbs and flat nails that are perfect for grasping and gathering fruit.

Regarding the extremities of the other species, herbivores possess hooves allowing them to walk easily about grassy plains, and carnivores possess sharp claws allowing them to violently attack their prey.

Tree-dwellers and fruit-gatherers also have stereoscopic binocular vision that makes vision precise enough to ascertain the position of tree limbs and objects—and only man has the intelligence to plant and harvest. Regarding food, man is most adept at gardening and being a caretaker of plants and orchards.

Among the various species throughout the animal world, the length of their particular alimentary canals also differs greatly in relation to their natural food. The gut of the carnivore is three times the length of the body, as they require a short, smooth, fast-acting gut since their natural flesh diet becomes quite toxic and cannot be retained within the intestine for long without poisonous putrefaction taking place.

The gut of the herbivore is sacculated and is 30 times the length of their body. Its herb and grass diet is coarse and fibrous, requiring longer digestion to break down cellulose. Likewise, the length of the omnivore's alimentary canal is generally 10 times its body trunk size. The gut of the frugivore (like man) is also sacculated and is 12 times the length of its body. (The length of the adult human alimentary canal is about 30 feet).

The human digestive tract is about four times as long as a carnivores. The intestine of the carnivore, is short and smooth in order to dissolve food rapidly and pass it quickly out of the system prior to the flesh putrefying. The human digestive tract is corrugated for the specific purpose of retaining food as long as possible, until all possible nutriment has been extracted—which is the *worst* possible condition for the digestion and processing of flesh foods.

Meat moves quickly through the carnivore's digestive tract and is quickly expelled, man's lengthy intestines cannot handle low-fiber foods (like meat and all other animal products) very quickly at all.

As a consequence, animal foods decrease the motility of the human intestine and putrefaction may occur, resulting in the release of many poisonous by-products as the low-fiber food moves ever so slowly. Eventual constipation develops as does cancer of the lower intestines (both of which are virtually unheard of on a high-fiber diet of raw fruits and vegetables).

Stomach form and size of the various animal species also vary markedly. In the carnivore, it is a small, round sack designed to dissolve flesh quickly and then pass it on for removal.

In plant eaters (particularly ruminants) stomachs are complicated adjoining sacks with ring-like convolutions. The frugivore stomach (including man) is oblong and is characterized by folds called *rugae* which serve to retain food for relatively long periods.

Organ sizes of various species also markedly vary. The liver and kidneys in the carnivore are larger than in vegetarian animals. A lion's kidney is twice the size of a bull's, and not much smaller than the elephant's. This allows the lion to handle large amounts of protein and nitrogenous waste products contained in its flesh-diet.

The carnivore's huge liver secretes larger amounts of bile into the small intestine than does the plant eater's liver. There is a direct relation between the quantity of meat eaten and the amount of bile secreted—and meat-eating therefore, places a strain on the small liver of humans which impairs the organ's function over a long period of time.

When you place man on a diet for which he is NOT naturally adapted, this places unnatural stress on his organs of purification and elimination.

Man has never adapted to the carnivorous diet that is high in animal products—man's liver is smaller than the carnivores and as a result, we cannot detoxify the poisonous products inherent within animal foods. Our kidneys are also smaller and become diseased from overwork caused by a diet high in animal protein.

The hydrochloric acid concentrations of various species are an additional determinant of their natural diet. A carnivore's gastric juice is highly acidic, serving to prevent putrefaction while flesh undergoes digestion.

Plant-eaters, however, (including man) secrete a much less concentrated and less abundant quantity of hydrochloric acid which does not curtail the bacterial decomposition of flesh—a process that begins at the animal's moment of death.

Flesh is digested in an acid medium within the stomach. Humans secrete a VERY weak concentration of hydrochloric acid relative to true carnivores, and little of the protein-splitting enzyme *pepsin* .

Carnivorous animals have concentrations of these flesh-digesting secretions 1100% greater than do humans. Lions can rip off and swallow your hand whole and quite readily digest it.

About 5% of the flesh volume of all animals consists of waste material called ***uric acid*** that is normally eliminated by the kidneys. Uric acid is a poison to humans because it is toxic and non-metabolizable. Nearly 100% of Americans suffer some form of osteoporosis which may be due, in large part, to the acidic end-products of meat-eating.

All carnivorous animals however, secrete the enzyme ***uricase*** which breaks down uric acid so it can be readily eliminated. Humans do not generate this enzyme—instead, we ABSORB uric acid when meat is eaten.

As a result, calcium urate crystals form and concentrate in joints, feet, and in the lower back. These deposits lead to arthritis, gout, rheumatism, bursitis, and lower back pain.

Humans are physiologically unsuited to utilizing meat as food. Natural carnivores swallow hunks of carrion almost unchewed, and the flesh is digested in the stomach with ease and facility. If humans were to do the same, we would digest very little of it before putrefaction set in and illness ensued. For humans, meat is a pathogenic and nutritionally deficient food.

The saliva pH of various species is another determinant of their natural diet. In carnivores, their saliva glands are small, and secrete an acid saliva having little or no effect on starch—which makes sense since flesh is virtually starch-free. Omnivores (like pigs) have tremendous salivary glands which secrete copious quantities of starch-splitting enzymes.

Humans only have one starch-splitting enzyme, versus a multitude of them in omnivores and natural starch-eating animals. Our *ptyalin* is very limited—this rules us out as being true graminivores (starch-eaters) which includes grains and cereals.

Frugivores (including man) have salivary glands that secrete alkaline saliva, containing only moderate amounts of ptyalin, which initiates starch digestion.

This tells us that humans and other frugivores can easily digest the small amount of starch contained in fresh fruits, nuts, and leafy greens—and that man is not intended to subsist on a diet of highly starchy foods as many currently do. (*Diabetes mellitus* is largely the result of consuming large amounts of refined sugars and starches. Even eating *predominantly* of whole grains and natural legumes as dietary staples can be injurious because of the need for excessive starch digestion).

Another anatomical comparison among species in the animal kingdom involves the structure of the skin. All vegetarian animals (including man) have abundant sweat glands.

In carnivores, however, their sweat glands are atrophied and inactive—they are exempt from profuse sweating in order to prevent a large fluid loss that would cause concentrated precipitation of nitrogenous wastes (from flesh-eating). This may also be why meat-eaters suffer in hot weather while vegetarians remain comfortable.

When humans started eating meat they did not over a period of thousands of years, develop fangs, claws or the concentrated hydrochloric acid solution which characterizes true carnivores. You need but examine the Eskimos who, perhaps, have eaten meat the longest, to confirm this. Animal species adapt very slowly to changed environmental conditions.

According to a continuous dietary study of 6,500 Chinese that began in 1983, nutritional biochemist T. Colin Campbell of Cornell University (who is also a member of the National Academy of Sciences), concluded that humans are still a vegetarian species, and that only in the last few thousand years have meat and animal products become staples of the Western diet. According to Dr. Campbell, "That's not nearly enough time to evolve new mechanisms to give us protection from these kinds of foods."

In summary, meat is not a suitable item of diet for humans for the following physiological reasons:

1. Flesh eating animals have a short intestine and bowel enabling them to rapidly expel the putrefactive flesh, while man has a long, complicated alimentary canal which enables plant nutrients to be slowly absorbed and assimilated;
2. Flesh eaters have a different type of intestinal bacterial flora than non-meat eaters (including man);
3. Flesh eaters have long sharp teeth, whereas man has the teeth of frugivores;
4. Man can grind his jaw, but flesh-eaters cannot—their jaws move vertically only;
5. Man sweats through his skin (as do other non-meat eaters such as horses, cows, monkeys, antelopes, etc.). whereas flesh-eaters sweat through their tongues;
6. Man sucks his liquids, whereas carnivores lap their liquids;
7. Man's saliva contains ptyalin (to commence starch digestion), whereas flesh-eaters have no ptyalin;
8. Flesh-eaters secrete 10 times the quantity of hydrochloric acid into the stomach than does man at a concentration much greater as well). This enables carnivores to cope with ingested bone, flesh, feathers, sinews, etc., since true meat-eaters take nourishment from practically the whole prey, not just muscle and selected organ meat as does man; and
9. Carnivores have large livers to aid in detoxifying the blood and to generate massive bile secretion, but man has a comparatively small liver.

Even ***psychologically***, we are not true carnivores. Natural meat-eaters stalk and pounce on their prey after overtaking it often with blinding bursts of speed. Carnivorous animals then sink their fangs deeply into its flesh, crushing and killing it. The food is then ripped to shreds, the bloody chunks swallowed with little mastication.

Humans are not natural killers, and do not psychologically savior these images, nor can they stomach eating raw the animal's blood, guts, bones, and organs.

Humans instead cook their meat, which literally means they are eating dead flesh because fire actually destroys living tissue. Cooked meat has no relation to live food or to the living flesh of an animal. Live plants, however, retain their form when picked for many days after. When they wilt, we do not eat them.

Our mental disposition matches our true dietary disposition. Our aesthetic standards attribute beauty to colorful fruit and shady trees, not to bleeding, dying animals. Contrary to learned, acquired perversions, we do not naturally savor flesh, blood, insects, or grasses (grains). We savor fruit.

In ascertaining our natural dietary equipment, you must envision us in a state of nature (rather than skyscrapers, freeways, and burger stands) where we once functioned totally with our natural equipment to acquire and eat foods. We were once tree-dwellers who lived upon fruits and nuts. Stoves, microwaves, toasters, pots and pans were not furnished as part of our natural equipment.

Are We Natural Vegetarians?

The biological equipment of humans is such that the body is most capable of obtaining complete and optimal nutrition from plant foods. **Actually, however, we are NOT true vegetarians either.** Natural herbivores (horses, cows, sheep, etc.) that subsist on green leaves and grasses (ruminants) have four stomachs containing special enzymes that can digest the carbohydrate *cellulose*, which is totally undigestible by humans.

Most of the calories of vegetables are bound within cellulose, whose fuel and nutrient value is largely unobtainable to our system (except for extremely valuable mineral matter from which our body does derive great benefit). True herbivores, however, are fully capable of attaining energy from herbs and grasses.

Unlike purely natural vegetarians in nature then, man's stomach cannot process large amounts of cellulose. Man cannot regurgitate and re-chew his food as does the cow. Nor can a man's stomach efficiently digest a mixture of all different types of foods as do true omnivores. Though anything in the world can be put into the human stomach and actually has, its physiology is such that only foods in compatible combinations can effectively be digested.

Frugivores are physiologically equipped to obtain energy primarily from the natural sugar in fruits. Humans are bestowed with a kind of "natural sweet tooth," to guide us in the selection of foods that meet our biological disposition and our caloric needs—namely, sweet juicy fruits.

Our anatomy is such that we are capable of picking fruits and to masticate, digest, and appropriate them with ease and efficiency. Fruits contain all the nutrients we need—vitamins, minerals, proteins (in the form of amino acids), fats, and carbohydrates.

Foods of our natural adaptation are the building blocks of balanced meals for humans. Fruits and succulent vegetables provide nutrients in proportion to the body's ability to utilize them. Our development in nature has occurred around the foods that best serve us—we adjusted so as to thrive on them.

Our physiological adaptations are so tailored that we can handle with ease and efficiency the proteins, fats and starches as they exist in fresh, ripe, raw fruits while receiving our *primary* energy needs—**caloric rich carbohydrates.**

The more foods to which we are adapted that we consume, the more nutrients we derive. Foods which we are biologically equipped to efficiently handle are readily digested and their nutrients swiftly absorbed. Fresh fruits and vegetables fill this bill ideally.

The bulk of most meals should consist of these foods for three main reasons: this prevents overeating concentrated foods; this insures an abundance of vitamins and minerals of the highest quality; and the needed bulk, necessary for normal peristalsis and elimination.

Our human structure attests that we are frugivores, as confirmed by the functions of the human body. Every alimentary function is geared to our fruitarian dietary.

Human saliva for instance, (in keeping with other frugivores) is alkaline which promotes carbohydrate digestion of fruit and initiates the neutralization of the incidental acids of many fruits—whereas the saliva of meat-eating animals is extremely acidic in order to digest concentrated protein and dissolve flesh with almost no mastication. Their rasping tongues also serve to tear flesh from bone, as compared to the smooth tongue of humans.

Man does not possess the physical apparatus that carnivores do for eating meat. Our teeth and the chemical makeup of our saliva and digestive juices point to a diet primarily of fruits and nonstarchy vegetables. The length of our small intestine is too long to handle putrefying meat, and is too short for grasses and grains. Humans instead are biologically adapted to eat a high-fiber, high-moisture diet to insure the health of our small and large intestines.

The most conclusive scientific evidence submitted, points to fruit as being the food of our biological adaptation. As seen from the viewpoint of comparative anatomy, man is a frugivore—man's digestive and other anatomical mechanisms are specifically adapted to fruits. This is denied by commercial interests, but an educated healthy populace would end their niche in the marketplace.

The Hygienic diet was not formulated on the basis of laboratory analyses of food or feeding experiments on rats. It is primarily based on a study of comparative anatomy and physiology that seeks to establish the biological class of animal to which man naturally belongs in order to determine his true dietary character.

No food could be more natural for us—as fruits even appeal to our visual, olfactory, and gustatory senses as well. Our natural diet should consist primarily of fruits, nuts, and green vegetables, as practically all animals in nature consume green foliage of some type. (Even the carnivore, at times, consumes large amounts of vegetation).

Green leafy plants may be regarded as a wild card throughout nature since whatever else an animal eats relative to their specific biological adaptations, some green leafy food is invariably included in the diet.

Health Requires Adherence to Our Biological Nature

Many different diets adequately provide all the nutrients required to sustain human life, yet the overall effect on health of these different diets varies drastically. This is why a healthful/optimum diet *cannot* be formulated solely on the basis of the nutritional analysis of food.

Food eaten must not only provide correct quantities and proportions of vital nutrients but also be well suited to the human digestive apparatus.

If a food contains abundant vitamins, minerals, and/or protein but also contains irritating substances toxic to the body, it cannot be regarded as a natural wholesome food for human consumption.

Incidentally, in nutrition the word ***"natural"*** DOES NOT mean that a particular food or substance comes from a plant or other source in nature, rather it means the foodstuff meets our biological needs and adaptations. Such "natural" plants, including tobacco, poppies, foxglove, belladona, poison ivy, etc., grow in nature but are deadly to humans. ***In relation to health, the term "natural" applies only insofar as it is natural to our well-being.***

Based upon man's digestive physiology, the following raw foodstuffs make up our natural diet (listed in order of preference relative to the food's biological value):

1. Fresh fruits
2. Succulent fruit-like vegetables (such as tomatoes)
3. Leafy greens and sprouts
4. Non-starchy vegetables
5. Nuts and seeds

The following foods, while not optimum, can be handled by man's digestive physiology in moderate amounts when properly combined:

1. Starchy vegetables
2. Grains and Cereals
3. Legumes

The following foods, while usually eaten on a vegetarian diet, are not well adapted to man's physiology and therefore place an undue strain on the organism:

1. Free oils
2. Dairy products

Finally, this last group of foods is definitely disruptive of man's health and are not compatible with our physiology:

1. Meat
2. Eggs
3. Cooked foods
4. Refined starches and sugars
5. Salt, herbs, spices, seasonings, dressings, etc.
6. All processed, preserved, fragmented, and artificial foods.

Those foods in the first list are most compatible with human physiology and those who desire optimum health should eat predominantly of these in moderate amounts, in proper combination. (Due to various anatomical and physiological weaknesses and defects that the body suffers over years of improper eating and living, not everyone can adhere to this dietary ideal with complete success, however, without first detoxifying the body. Even then, the diet should be tailored to individual needs).

If we wish to achieve the highest level of health to which our potential permits, we *must* respect our natural adaptations and our biological heritage.

You would never expect deer, cattle, or other herbivores to thrive on anything except grass, as this is their adaptation. **A living organism is what it is in nature and cannot act contrary to its nature while striving to maintain a healthful state—*and this fact is equally true for mankind.***

Our adaptation is to a diet made up of mostly fruits, vegetables, nuts, and certain edible seeds. We serve ourselves best by observing our natural dietary needs.

Food is man's most immediate contact with nature. As such, it must be suited to the laws that govern our body, otherwise the body breaks down. The very structure and function of the body—its physiological and biological methods, its capacities and limitations—dictate certain unchanging principles which in turn dictate in what manner the human organism must be nourished in order to remain in superb health.

By our very nature we cannot function properly contrary to this mandate without major compromises to health and the manifestation of abnormal (although prevalent) chronic disease.

While the human body is remarkably flexible, it cannot adapt in the long run to foods that are beyond the limits of our digestive enzymes or that have been radically altered from their natural form without major health deterioration and premature aging taking place.

To build health we must adopt more scientifically accurate and biologically appropriate ways of eating and living. At first, these changes may seem strange but only because our former habits and beliefs were based on false theories and entirely erroneous notions *whose motives are profit for food manufacturers and not health for consumers.*

While circumstances and conditions may vary, the principles of nutrition are NOT subject to change. All humans are fundamentally alike with similar organs, cells, and tissues which may vary in efficiency but not in their method of function. Nature provides all that man (and every species) requires to live in health.

Human needs are most fully and completely met so long as our biological needs are fulfilled. By using nature's food packages, health is most easily achieved (provided that other requisites of well-being are likewise attended to).

When our species conforms to the laws of our very nature, the human organism prospers. To develop *optimum* health, man must eat of mostly those foods designed specifically for his structural and functional requirements, and must eat them relatively whole, without alteration of any kind.

Animal products, decaying and fermented foods, and inorganic elements cannot be eaten without causing damage to the body. Cooking also pathologically alters food as heat chemically changes it and returns molecules to a largely unusable inorganic state.

Foods must be eaten that are designed specifically to satisfy our structural and functional requirements—and these need to be ingested without alteration of any kind.

The closer the food is eaten as yielded by field and orchard, the more it is fit to support life. Compromises result in compromised health and longevity. In no area of life do we flaunt our biological disposition so flagrantly as in our dietary practices. Food is our area of greatest deviation from our natural norms.

Forty-five percent of the average American's caloric intake consists of fats that have been fried, refined, denatured, and rendered carcinogenic. Animal products make up a substantial amount of the American diet.

Cooked foods (all of which beget leucocytosis), poisonous habits (including drugs, alcohol, caffeine, smoking, condiments, etc.) all contribute to pathology and destruction of health. Mankind cannot partake of such nutritionally antagonistic "foods" to which he is not well adapted and maintain a long healthy life.

The key to a perpetual state of well-being is biologically correct living practices. Our eating habits in particular should be determined by our physiological adaptations. Animals in nature live in accord with their biological heritage and eat according to their natural diet. They do not develop chronic disease—they live out their normal lifespan and die a relatively peaceful, painless, natural death.

Humans, by and large, have strayed from their natural diet and for this reason, regularly suffer chronic disease and early death. Consider, for example, that America consumes less than 10% of its correct fruitarian diet. In addition, since the bulk of America's fruit is consumed by less than 25% of our populace, it should be no surprise that there is such a great preponderance of disease among us.

All transgressions of our natural diet have pathological results whether evident or not. The body functions perfectly within the context of its natural dietary needs and other important vital health practices.

The causes of bodily disease are multiple, and are related to all the various facets of our existence—nutrition, exercise, rest, mental and emotional factors, relationships with others, our philosophical and spiritual well-being, etc. The most significant causes however, are those related to our most fundamental biological needs (food, shelter, etc.). Those relating to our mental and emotional life complete the picture.

Within modern society, most causes of disease are within the total control of the individual. By taking control of our life and applying self-management that is based on biologically proven facts, health is built.

Optimum levels of well-being can only be achieved by living in accordance with the innate dictates of our human physiology. Humans who adhere to their natural diet and observe the other modalities of healthful living, can expect to live to a healthy, ripe old age and pass on naturally.

True, we can eat anything we wish, this is man's free choice. If you are satisfied with the ordinary low level of health "enjoyed" by modern civilized mankind, then dietary change is difficult.

Good health is not merely the absence of symptoms and pain, rather optimum health produces marked improvements in our physical, mental, emotional, and spiritual facets of living such that it becomes a joy to live according to our system's actual needs.

Living healthfully means observing our physiological mandate. The body is fully self-operating and self-sufficient if its needs are furnished. Basically, these needs are foods to which we are biologically adapted, relatively pure air and water, adequate rest and sleep, vigorous physical activity, sunshine, recreation and play, emotional poise, security of life, love, and self-mastery.

We should put into our body *only* pure (distilled) water, fresh air, sunlight, and a diet predominating in fresh, raw fruit with a moderate amount of fresh, raw vegetables, nuts, and seeds. Eat foods to which our body is intended to function most normally and ideally on, plus follow the other essential needs of living and the majority of our ailments will largely be a thing of the past.

SECTION III

THE SOLUTION IN THEORY AND PRACTICE:

NATURAL HYGIENE— THE TRUE *SELF* HEALTH CARE SYSTEM

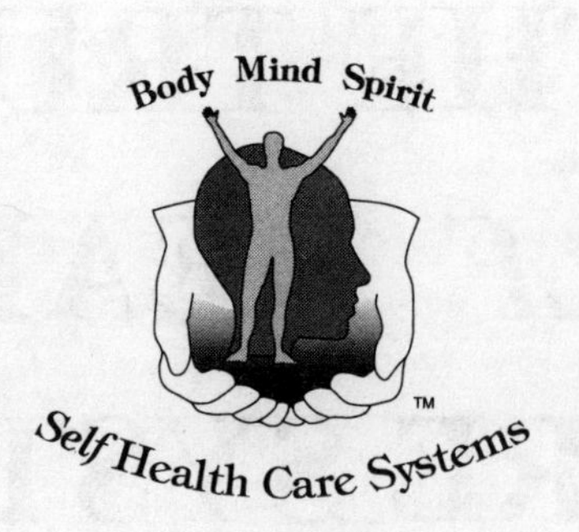
Body Mind Spirit
Self Health Care Systems
™

Chapter 8

THE PHILOSOPHY AND IMPLEMENTATION OF HOLISTIC HEALTH CARE

Nearly 6,000 years ago on a pyramid that has been dated to 3800 B.C., the following inscription was laid: *"Man lives on one-quarter of what he eats. On the other three-quarters, lives his doctor."*

Natural Hygiene is not *merely* a dietary system, but is a total way of life—it is not a complex of cures for disease, but is a complete plan of living. Self Health Care needs to be applied where violations of the human norm are most striking. This area happens to be what we eat.

For health to be truly established as a permanent feature of life, a complete well-rounded program of living is essential. Health can only be produced and maintained as a wholeness, and the total health care system must meet all the requisites of our well-being.

The Practical Application of Natural Hygiene

The practical application of Natural Hygiene consists of many practices that, collectively, comprise biologically correct living. Specifically:

FOOD

DO

- Eat predominantly of fresh raw fruits, vegetables, nuts and seeds;
- Eat predominantly of raw, live food;
- Learn and apply the rules of food combining to insure efficient and easy digestion;
- Eat foods at room temperature;
- Chew thoroughly to maximize surface area of the food for complete digestion;
- Eat when relaxed; and
- Eat only when hungry.

DON'T

- Cook or overcook food—past 120 degrees, nutrients are destroyed;
- Overeat;
- Eat when emotionally unsettled when tired when in pain or immediately after hard physical work;
- Salt or overly season foods; or
- Eat many strong-tasting foods including hot peppers, garlic, onions, mustard, etc.

WATER

DO

- Drink only distilled (soft) water;
- Drink only when thirsty; and
- Drink only enough to quench thirst.

DON'T

- Drink with your meals.

AIR

DO

- Get as much fresh air as possible;
- Allow for maximum ventilation when indoors;
- Walk on streets that have less vehicular traffic and exhaust; and
- Make sure indoor air is free of sprays, circulating dust, etc.

DON'T

- Breathe through your mouth;
- Inhale tobacco smoke;
- Permit smoking in your home or office; or
- Breathe excessively cold air (if possible).

PHYSICAL ACTIVITY

DO

- Exercise vigorously;
- Involve all parts of the body, preferably exercising the muscles against resistance; and
- Exercise in fresh air (or if indoors, with windows open).

DON'T

- Exercise to the point of exhaustion;
- Exercise immediately following a meal;
- Prolong muscular contractions beyond a few seconds; and
- Breathe deeply without simultaneously remaining active.

REST

DO

- Cease activity sometime during the day by napping or meditating;
- Close the eyes; and
- Rest when tired.

DON'T

- Read or watch television while resting.

SLEEP

DO

- Go to bed early;
- Select a dark, quiet, well ventilated room; and
- Maintain a comfortable body temperature.

DON'T

- Eat before retiring.

LIGHT AND SUNSHINE

DO

- Expose as much of your skin to sunlight as possible, up to an hour maximum daily;
- Use natural, not artificial light (rays penetrate only white or light colored porous clothing); and
- In cold climates, while indoors, get sunlight through open windows with heater turned on to avoid undue chilling.

DON'T

- Remain in sunlight for long periods; or
- Expose yourself to the midday sun;

EMOTIONAL WELL-BEING

DO

- Find something about which to be happy everyday;
- Feed your emotions daily with inspirational thoughts, pleasant sights and sounds, kind words and the like;
- Keep negative emotions to a minimum; and
- Couple negative emotions (fear, grief, anger, depression, etc.) with physical activity.

DON'T

- Dwell on the negative.

TEMPERATURE

DO

- Maintain a comfortable temperature at all times; and

DON'T

- Take excessively hot or cold baths.

CLOTHING

DO

- Wear clothes of porous material (cotton); and
- Wear light-colored clothing.
- Dress for comfort, not merely for fashion.

DON'T

- Wear synthetic clothing; or
- Wear constricting clothing (girdles, tight belts, etc.).

POSTURE

DO

- Sit erect at all times; and
- Keep your head straight-up while walking, standing, or sitting.

ZEST FOR LIVING

DO

- Pursue some constructive objective; and
- Engage in some activity which gives you fulfillment.

Natural Hygiene does not substitute foods, fasting, sunbathing, etc., for drugs, but it uses these influences because they are essentials of health. Hygienic Health Care peddles no cures and recognizes none. Instead, only *nature*, meaning those normal influences and processes of life, restores health.

Hygienic Self-Health Care cannot be reduced to a series of rules and regulations that involve *absolute* terms like "always" and "never." Each day, however, all of us have to make decisions about how we will live in such a way that we remain comfortable and relaxed with our lifestyle—and not uptight or fanatical.

While there are no quick and easy answers to many of our challenges, when situations arise where the ideal choice is not available, then make the next best choice. Natural Hygiene is not a rigid code of behavior—rather, it is a flexible system of Self-Health Care that allows life to be lived to its fullest while being adapted to individual needs.

And it is much more than a system of trivial, minor restraints. Those who believe that a Hygienic lifestyle is limited, boring and yields little joy are many times themselves irritable, constipated, suffer frequent headaches and indigestion, and are enslaved to desires that are never satisfied.

They may feel "free" from discipline but, as a result, they frequently suffer aches and pains, weakness, misery, fears, and inner conflicts since their health and destiny seems out of their hands.

Power comes by discipline to our natural mandate, and lack of it dissipates strength and life itself. Does this enslave us? Hardly. On the contrary, we are freed from cravings for alcohol, drugs, excessive sexual stimulation, uncontrolled appetite, overeating, and pain from a weakened body. The disciplined Hygienist is free to do whatever he or she likes in knowing that prudent, conscious living harmonizes us with our essential nature.

Sacrifices are not sacrifices when they help us achieve a worthy goal—namely, a life without suffering and the maintenance of our faculties, which enabling us to pursue pleasurable endeavors.

In this regard, we must refrain from thinking of Natural Hygiene as a system of mere restrictions and instead, lift it to a plane whereby it guides and challenges us as a means to achieve a more abundant and higher quality of health and well-being.

Hygienic methods accord to nature the conditions and the opportunity to rebuild health. Only in nature exists the power of healing. Hygienic Self-Health Care presents an educational program that provides knowledge of harmonious living in tune with our natural disposition, and is a system based on personal responsibility.

Health is a natural, inalienable right and its attainment is dependent on knowledge, and then consistently acting on what has been learned in order to provide the basic needs of organic existence while simultaneously avoiding that which is contrary to our systemic needs.

How do we know what life's requirements are and what we need to avoid? The very thrust of Natural Hygiene lies in the simple message that to create and maintain health, all we need is to live in accord with our biological heritage by providing those influences and elements which, as a creature of nature, mankind has been dependent upon during our millions of years of development.

This means assuring ourselves of adequate fresh air, pure water, wholesome food in its natural unaltered state to which humans are constitutionally adapted, moderate sunshine, sufficient rest and sleep, exercise, maintenance of body warmth, internal and external cleanliness of the body, security of life and its means, pleasant environment, creative useful work, belonging to a friendly social group, love, indulgence of our aesthetic senses, healthy expression of the reproductive instinct, and most notably, self-mastery.

Natural Hygiene holds that deprivation of these factors and influences or any interference with them, are necessarily detrimental to human well-being.

Natural Hygiene studies and understands precisely the nature of air, water, food, sunlight, exercise, rest, sleep, temperature, clothing, housing, emotions, etc., relative to the preservation of health and advocates the constant application of this knowledge daily in accordance with our systemic needs.

A well-rounded, fully integrated system of Self-Health Care necessarily includes ALL the conditions of health and not one that focuses attention on diet, exercise, or emotional poise alone. Health must be based on the *total* mode of living and be built and maintained as a unit, and not in a fragmented, piece-meal manner.

Hygienic Self-Health Care is in total accord with the laws of physiology as expressed in the realm of biology. The food it employs, the exercise it requires, the rest it enforces, the sunshine it utilizes, and the abstinence required are all implemented with regard to the natural requirements of the body and not in relation to some suppose need to *"cure"* disease.

The selection and administration of Hygienic means are totally governed by the human constitution and the laws of its actions and reactions.

This philosophy of health holds as its basic tenets that:

1. Robust health is the NORMAL state of human existence and is realizable without interruption throughout the entire life span;
2. Only through nature, which developed human beings to such a high state over millions of years of evolution, can solutions to the mysteries of disease, suffering and premature death be found;
3. All physical maladies represent ABNORMAL body conditions that are unnecessary and avoidable;
4. Only by living naturally—by aligning ourselves with our biological heritage—can humans achieve their highest potential for health and well-being; and
5. All humans should be splendidly developed and as functionally sound as the deer of the fields and animals of the forests. All humans, basically, should be a standard of beauty and physical excellence.

In addition, Natural Hygiene recognizes the following fundamental principles:

- That the human body when supplied with its basic needs, is a completely self-sufficient organism with inherent abilities capable of maintaining itself in high-level functioning for the duration of its life potential, perhaps a minimum of 120 years;
- That almost all diseases are caused by bodily abuse, or by failure to live in accord with our biological needs;
- That in the event of sickness, the body requires only the removal of causes of malfunction to restore itself to health. **The body under normal circumstances, is completely self-correcting and self-healing;**
- Our physiological requirements in illness are no different than when in a state of health, except that an ailing body requires complete physiological rest in order for its restorative, regenerative, and healing capabilities to function unhampered and unimpeded;
- There must always be a normal connection between the living organism (whether in a state of health or disease) and the materials that contribute to sustain biological and physiological phenomena. In other words, ***any substance or process that is toxic or unusable in a state of health, is equally unusable in disease;***
- All processes of recovery and healing are but extensions and modifications of the processes that preserve health. All materials and processes employed in caring for the sick must be compatible with sustaining life in a healthful state; and, finally,
- In all states of impaired health (acute or chronic illness and when injured), the physiological requirements of life—namely, air, water, food, sunlight, activity, temperature, rest, sleep, etc.—must be supplied solely in keeping with the ability of the body to appropriate and use them.

The SCIENCE of Holistic Health Care vs. the Profitization of Commercial Health Care

Although Natural Hygiene originated almost two centuries ago, it has taken until now to develop into a truly scientific healing system. Natural Hygiene is indeed a scientific study since its basis is strictly in accord with our biological disposition.

Hygienic Health Care encompasses all that bears upon health, be it physical, mental, social, ecological, economic, or spiritual. Health and disease are not accidents nor do they develop by chance—rather, they evolve from the laws of cause and effect.

Just as the law of gravity carries a balloon upward as well as back to the earth; or floats a ship under one set of conditions and sinks it under another; and just as the same laws of chemistry that preserves dynamite under one set of conditions and explodes it under another; so to do laws of physiology produce health under one set of conditions and disease under another.

Knowledge and application of these physiological laws makes health and disease a matter of choice, depending on the conditions we supply. In this sense, living "scientifically" means living in accord with our biological heritage.

Science is defined as the systematic observation of natural phenomena for the purpose of discovering general underlying laws that govern these phenomena. In this way, we apply these same principles and shape our environment to make life easier or more comfortable.

The Hygienic Health Care System in both conditions of health and illness involves the application of scientific principles of biology to the varying circumstances of life. ***Hygienic methods are not experimental and are not haphazard—*** rather, Hygiene rests upon the immutable principles that govern the physiology of the human being and is established on fixed laws of nature which guide the employment of all its measures.

In other words, Natural Hygiene is based on demonstrable principles of health and not on trial and error. Application of these principles in life leads to the production of the desired salubrious state.

The laws of our being and the principles of science are just as certain, fixed, and immutable in their relation to health and disease, as they are in relation to everything else studied by science whether in physics, astronomy, chemistry, mathematics or what have you. Natural Hygiene involves the exploration and implementation of those elements and influences that can be invoked to exalt our lives and well-being.

Certain scientific principles are applicable to human welfare. Studying and systematizing these such that life may benefit from them is the aim of Hygienic Health Care. In this sense, scientific knowledge becomes personal and relevant to all facets of living. Contrarily, science today is mostly impersonal, impractical, and hardly of benefit to daily living *except* to those who profit by exploiting the environment and the world's masses.

Scientific study of any kind, whether through books or by direct personal experience, cannot be divorced from our daily affairs and remain of value to our well-being. Rather than studying the science of health, modern medicine has studied the laws of disease. Because mankind has not **APPLIED** the study of physiology and of Hygiene to lifestyle, we have fallen victim to our biological indiscretions.

The practical aspect of Natural Hygiene encompasses the techniques that have been learned from studying natural laws that determine health. The more these techniques and guidelines are applied in daily living, the more they enhance the quality and quantity of our life.

Natural Hygiene is based on Nature. All the answers are there for us to discover and benefit from. Humans have existed for millions of years without published research and guiding documentation to determine the correctness of their lifestyle. Unfortunately, today's fashion is such that unless a sterling truth proceeds directly from a laboratory or from a "credentialed" authority, it is detested, scoffed at, and deemed unworthy of acceptance.

There are few who will not swallow without question every pronouncement that proceeds from our highly regarded "scientists" who, more often than not, are funded by industries with vested interests in obtaining biased research results to substantiate whatever product and/or service they are selling.

But how was the value of food verified before the advent of laboratories? How was it learned that warmth and sunlight are beneficial? How was air discovered to be a necessity?

Natural Hygiene exists as part of our inherent nature, for it is instinctual and perpetual regardless of intellectual rejection, or the mental masturbation of our so-called scholars and experts. Our intellects *are not* too frail to ascertain and verify the facts for ourselves by applying nature's principles in our own lives.

The Hygienic Health Care system has no products to sell and no vested interest to serve. People unfortunately tend to think that what works in this world must be complicated, sophisticated, and born out of the minds of "experts"—and this is why the truth regarding health, even though simple, is often rejected.

Natural Hygiene, however, is in harmony with nature; in

accord with the principles of vital organic existence; correct in science; sound in philosophy and ethics; in agreement with common sense; and successful in its results.

To down play principles of Natural Hygiene merely because they were formulated or discovered years ago is as ridiculous as casting aside Newton's Law of Gravity because IT was discovered years ago. The passage of time does not invalidate principles of science or the value of knowledge.

Few people realize that among the oldest and most respected educational institutions in this country, many are not "accredited." Harvard and other Ivy League schools are examples, founded and established well before accreditation was implemented as a way for special interests, through the vehicle of government, to monopolize and control curricula in this country.

Look at it this way, if accredited schools of nutrition had answers, why is this country so confused about what to eat in order to generate health and so obsessed with losing weight? Why do millions purchase diet books and enter diet centers? Why are eating habits so poor in this country, especially in public schools where a huge percentage of our country's poorer children receive their meals each day?

Meals in our public schools that are formulated by the American Dietetic Association are so overloaded with fat that they literally ooze with grease. Junk foods, vending machines, sodas and chips are the staple in our public schools because "they are profitable" we are told by administrators.

Why don't credentialed ADA dietitians do something about this appalling situation by promoting programs that are in line with recommendations of the National Academy of Sciences, the National Cancer Institute, and the American Heart Association which advise eating *far* more fresh fruits and vegetables, reducing fat and cholesterol, and cutting

back on high-salt, high-sugar, and processed foods?

Most of those who emphasize credentials are apparently interested in maintaining the status quo—and it appears power is their main concern, not people. What really counts is *results* in people's lives, not a framed certificate or the letters "Ph.D" tacked on to one's name. After all, take a look around at the current state of affairs in health care. With all our knowledgeable "experts," we are sure in a sorry state.

As a profession, many licensed Hygienic practitioners practice under the guise of medical science, chiropractic, naturopathy or some other healing art (see appendix C for listings). Many have dropped the drugging methods of medicine and have undergone internships under the auspices of those adept in the practical application of Hygienic fasting.

This state of affairs is undesirable, however, since it severely limits the number of Hygienic Health Care practitioners to a very small number—**but this does not prevent the majority of people from applying Hygienic Self-Health Care into their own lives, for its safety and simplicity make it an effective tool in the hands of the layman.**

Natural Hygiene is simple, easily understood, and readily applicable to life. A little understanding goes a long way, and a firm grasp of the most salient principles is of more benefit than mastering the intricate data pertaining to modern nutrition. Once the knowledge of Hygienic Health Care becomes widespread, it would be self-applied (with rare exceptions in the severely debilitated).

The present need for a large number of professional Hygienic practitioners would then disappear, and the profession would remain only on a small scale primarily as educators of a biologically-adapted lifestyle and to help people become self-reliant in matters of health.

Natural Hygiene Practitioners EDUCATE—and DO NOT Cure or Treat Disease

Both licensed and non-licensed Hygienic Health Care practitioners are *educators* who teach, guide and counsel others in matters of health. In no way, shape, or form do they diagnose, prescribe, or treat disease. They follow no course of therapy but, instead, TEACH people how to build health through biologically healthful living.

For the body to constantly strive towards health, obstacles must be minimized. The role of the Hygienic practitioner is to educate their clients to remove obstacles by living biologically adapted lifestyles ensuring that the conditions for health are supplied in proper quantity and quality.

Hygienic practitioners can *only* educate and can in no way change the lifestyle of anyone. If the education is not applied in daily living, disease continues to occur.

Hygienic Health-Care is not a cure or treatment—it is a way of life. If not implemented, this does not signify a failure of Hygiene, but rather a failure of the individual to live in accord with his or her biological needs.

To repeat, hygienic practitioners DO NOT heal, cure, treat, or give drugs. Hygienists bathe the body ***to cleanse it*** , and not to treat disease; they feed and sunbathe the body ***to nourish it*** , and not to cure disease; they recommend exercise ***to meet everyday needs for physical activity*** , and not as a remedy; they secure rest as a means of ***recuperation*** , and not to heal illness; they advise fasting as a means of ***physiological rest to enhance self-healing*** , and not as a curative; they cultivate mental poise as means of ***conserving energy*** , and not as psychotherapy; and they suggest the cessation of lifestyle habits that are contrary to our biological mandate as a way of **avoiding**

energy drain and as a way of avoiding injury, and not as a therapeutic agent.

Natural Hygiene as Applied to Disease

The work of the hygienic practitioner is that of caring for the WHOLE human organism, not of treating any fictional disease entity.

Many people think of Hygienic agencies as limited in their work only to the preservation of health—while good for the person who is well, Hygiene is erroneously believed to be too weak and unreliable when diseased. After all, when ill don't we need potent, powerful medicine?

Getting along when sick WITHOUT medicine sounds strange when we first hear of it, since the idea of caring medicinally for the sick is deeply ingrained in us from day one.

History reveals, however, that the theory of the earth revolving on its axis was denied for *1,200 years* before finally being accepted. In like manner, it is difficult for people to accept that Hygienic agents—those solely adapted to health—are better for the sick than are pathogenic agents—those that induce sickness in those who are well.

Hygiene when applied to the sick consists of finding and removing the causes of suffering and restoring the conditions of a healthy life. This is accomplished through education—the teaching of how to prepare and eat a biologically proper diet; how to secure fresh air in abundance; how to exercise and secure adequate sunshine; and down the line through the essentials of health.

Hygienic Health Care is a system of purification and rejuvenation which uses agents that are normal to the body in order to cleanse and restore the system to a salubrious state. **The essence of *Natural Hygiene Self-Health Care* is "remove the cause, and the effect will cease"**—remove the causes of disease and the body will heal itself. Fasting, resting, exercise, and sunshine restore the body's ability to normalize its metabolic function.

Hygienic care of the sick involves the removal of the cause of illness such that the individual does not continue to build a state of toxemia. Hygienic care is not mere palliation, that is, mere suppression of symptoms. Rather, it removes causes and initiates healthful practices. So long as Hygienic living is implemented, the diseased condition does not recur.

To a large extent the body protects itself—but even constant drops of water can wear away stone. Any program of health care that does not remove the causes of illness, will not generate health, for if the need for the disease/purification process is not removed, lasting health will not ensue. **To identify and remove the causes of disease is the constant aim of Hygiene Self-Health Care.**

In addition to implementing Hygienic instruction, we also must understand the underlying mechanics of these fundamental principles. Understanding the parts of an automobile enables us to understand what to do when it malfunctions, as well as what is essential to maintain it in proper working order.

Similarly, with the human constitution—to know the means whose legitimate use keeps health preserved and life prolonged, is also to know the means necessary to restore health when sick. To restore health by those same essentials of life that keep us in a salubrious state in the first place is to know what is required to re-establish wellness.

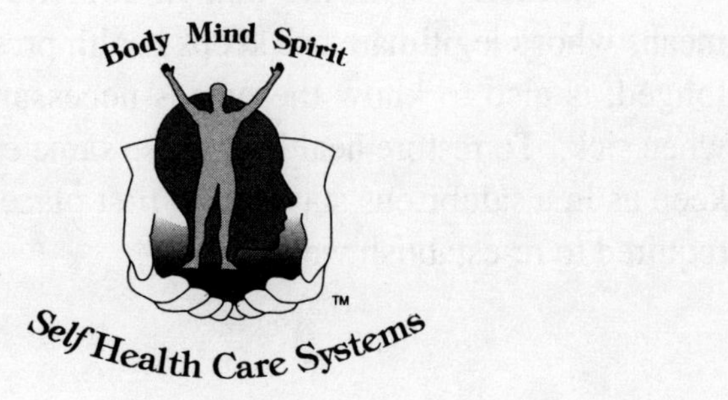
Body Mind Spirit
TM
Self Health Care Systems

Chapter 9

REDEFINING HEALTH AND DISEASE

Hygienic Self-Health Care, in comparison to modern medicine, offers a unique view of the very nature of health and disease. Health is defined by *Dorlands Medical Dictionary* as a state of optimal function of our physical, mental, and social well-being—not merely the an absence of disease symptoms.

In actual medical practice, however, health *is* commonly defined by absence of disease symptoms. Even if symptoms DO manifest, but not much worse than the norm as seen in other patients, the physician may still pronounce you healthy—a kind of health by default, if you will.

Modern medicine defines disease as the abnormal degeneration or death of cellular tissue mainly due to invasion by bacterial or viral microorganisms, as well as the processes preceding the degeneration, including fever, headache, inflammation, vomiting, diarrhea, etc.

Hygienists and those who study health realize this is a serious misconception since the **self**-healing mechanism of the body produces these natural processes as needed to restore homeostatic balance and prevent damage to the system.

According to Natural Hygiene, disease is caused by violating our biological nature. Hygienic Self-Health Care stops these violations and, instead, resupplies the conditions of health.

Health and disease are *not* opposite conditions but are varying expressions of the same underlying continuum of physiology whose manifestations are dependent on the system's internal and external state.

Health is an ideal physiological state of body and mind where our emotions are predominantly peaceful, and our organs all work in harmony. Health is a state of vitality that is generated solely by the human organism when its requisite needs are consistently furnished, and when levels of stress do not exceed the body's inherent capacities to cope.

Disease represents any departure from this ideal. In other words, health manifests because of *normal* conditions, while disease manifests because of *abnormal* conditions. Simply put, disease is abnormal, vital action.

Disease is as much a vital process as is health. Whereas health is vital action involving the **normal, physiological renewal** and conservation of bodily organs, disease is vital action in defense and reparation of these organs under **abnormal, pathological conditions.**

Whereas *health* involves processes that nourish, replenish, and develop the body's organic structures by converting food into tissue, *disease* involves the expulsion of accumulated wastes, as well as the necessary remedial processes required to repair damaged tissues. While the body in times of disease utilizes the same powers that are active in health, these are redirected in defending the organism against injurious or abnormal conditions.

Acute disease is a vital process of purification and repair, it is not an enemy of the body but is a struggle of the system in self-defense against poisonous toxins that have accumulated—called **toxicosis**—which forms the actual cause of disease.

Toxemia and the "Polluted Body"—the Root Cause of Disease

The root cause of disease is **systemic toxemia**, literally meaning a "polluted body," one overly saturated with metabolic wastes, chemicals, and poisons.

Toxemia is a poisoned condition of the organism where over-accumulated waste materials inhibit the body's efficient, normal metabolic functioning. Toxicosis implies a disturbance in homeostasis—the accumulation of toxic metabolic by-products in the body's blood and tissues.

Disease is a pathological process of physiological and biochemical changes within the body caused by internal toxicity. Disease is the result of enervation—as our energy reserves become bankrupt, our energy levels decrease and the body's functional efficiency deteriorates. We slowly evolve into a state of toxicosis, where the body is saturated with toxic matter.

We do not die from acute disease since disease is the body's normal response to a state of internal emergency. Rather, we die from toxemia and its causes.

The causes of toxemia and enervation are largely exogenous—from outside the body. Toxemia may be due to metabolic waste accumulating as a result of exhaustion, or from absorbing poisons from our environment such as improper foods, stimulants, drugs, preservatives, metals, insecticides, or toxic gases.

Major causes of toxemia include those habits of living that either fail to supply our most fundamental biological needs or that exceed our physiological limitations—too much food; too much food that we are not biologically equipped to metabolize; insufficient rest and sleep; insufficient exercise, and so on, all of which produce internal stresses and a chemical burden the body cannot handle. Likewise, toxic conditions result from years of improper living, biologically incorrect eating, taking drugs, chemicals, and other foreign substances.

Acute Disease is a Self-Initiated "House-Cleaning" of the Body

The body itself institutes the acute disease process in order to clean the system of internal toxic matter. Such "housecleaning" is initiated when body integrity is compromised or threatened by poisonous accumulations.

Acute illness represents an emergency measure on the body's behalf to rid itself of an intolerable condition brought upon by the errors and omissions inherited in unconscious "civilized living." Disease originates in the body as a result of poor eating and living habits including physical, mental, and emotional practices which subtly weaken the organism by insidiously draining our energy.

Poisonous substances and influences that the body experiences regularly in the standard American lifestyle include overeating; overconsumption of refined, manufactured carbohydrates; TOO FEW fresh uncooked fruits, and vegetables; insufficient muscular activity; consuming animal products, coffee, tea, soft drinks, junk foods, alcohol, and drugs etc.; not enough clean fresh air; insufficient rest, and sleep; excessive stress, overwork, sexual excess; tension, worry, depression; impure water, cooked food, sugar, salt, caffeine, tobacco, serum injections, and so on. All of these contribute to cellular contamination which eventually builds disease.

The bodies of most people take so much punishment

during the time of infancy (from formula feeding, vaccinations, improper foods, etc.), that their bloodstream quickly becomes contaminated and retains toxic material as their level of toleration gradually increases. As this continues, the child develops fewer eliminative crises and the body is forced to live with internal poisons.

The net result of "civilized living" is that the blood and blood vessels are often filled with waste material. The body suffers from toxemia, and health declines. Over long periods, the body's natural defenses weaken, such that it is no longer capable of proper and thorough healing.

A toxic state of the body develops slowly and devitalizes our tissues for years, resulting in delayed healing and degeneration in injured or devitalized areas. When we live in a manner to maintain a continuous toxic state, we are in line for developing any disease to which systemic weakness and/or environment determines.

According to the body's predilection, the toxic system may express its plight as any of numerous diseases each with its particular set of symptoms. These are desperate measures on the part of the organism to throw off the accumulated wastes or to cope with impaired conditions.

All diseases are the result of a polluted body—a body laden with morbid material which threatens body integrity. The manner and location in which the body elects to purify itself determines the symptomology involved and earns many different names such as asthma, headaches, influenza, etc.

For instance, if the body selects the respiratory tract, a cold, flu, sinusitis, or bronchitis may develop. ONLY the body has the integrated power, resources, intelligence, and unity of purpose to accomplish this.

The body concentrates its remedial action where toxins have been stored and concentrated, and where their removal is imminent. This is a process of self-healing as the body acts in its best interest to purify, cleanse, and reconstruct damaged cells and tissues.

Body Vitality Determines the Intensity of Disease

The level of toxic overload and the residual vitality of the individual also determines the location and the type of disease crisis. When we are young, our body is vital and the return to health occurs vigorously with speed and efficiency. When we get older, the return to health may be elusive as the body's reparative mechanisms slowly lose their ability to mend the system.

An infant, for instance, with his or her pure body and high vitality, tolerates only a very low level of toxicity. Colds are frequent and illness usually violent.

Elderly people, however, with a lifetime of toxins in their body and with low vitality generally have fewer colds and acute illnesses. The body CANNOT conduct defensive disease-/healing crises if its vitality has been lowered to the point where it no longer has the energy and resources to initiate and conduct extraordinary detoxification.

Because so few older people maintain a vital body, their toxic overload drags them down into chronic disease. "Unexpected death" or "sudden onset of cancer" all too commonly occurs.

When body vitality is high (as in children) acute disease symptoms can be very violent. But if vitality is low (as in the elderly) symptoms may be mild or will become chronic. Outward manifestation of disease is always dependent upon the body's existing vitality; its systemic weaknesses; and the amount and type of impurities present in the system.

The body's vitality (its level of strength) or weakness depends entirely upon its nerve energy reserves since all functions of the body are carried out according to the amount of energy generated and distributed via the nervous system. When nerve energy is not equal to the demands of the body, organic functioning is impaired, resulting in the retention of waste material which produces toxemia.

Overwork, worry, inadequate rest and sleep, and overstimulation short-circuit and drain our energy supply, with the consequence of being enervated. This weakened state expresses itself in imperfect elimination, and the **IN**ability of the body to rid itself of metabolic waste products which then brings on autotoxemia—a state of self-poisoning.

Unhygienic conditions of life give rise to a toxic state of the body. Toxicosis (a saturation of poisons) eventually develops beyond a point of vital toleration and evokes extraordinary eliminative efforts—the healing crisis called "disease."

To overcome toxemia, the body suspends or reduces certain physical actions such as digestion and muscular effort in order to conserve energy and nerve function. These vital resources are then re-directed to create quantitative physiological changes throughout the body, to produce such actions as fever, diarrhea, polyuria (frequent urination), vomiting, etc., to remove irritating agents and detoxify the system.

Such actions reflect the coordinated efforts of a complex, intelligent organism. Recognizing disease as the "cure," why employ drugs to stop the curative process? This only works AGAINST the body's efforts to heal.

The body constantly protects itself but cannot do so indefinitely just as constant drops of water wear away stone. Any program of care that does not remove the causes of toxemia does not generate health, for the body does not cease to generate disease over the long haul until either its success or death terminates the effort. If the need for disease is not removed, health will not ensue.

We cannot indulge in the causes of disease and

expect to be free of its consequences—physiology does not work that way. We cannot be made exempt from violations of the laws of health.

Most disease is autogenerated. Excluding those acts of poisoning by externally ingested toxic substances and iatrogenic (medically caused) disease, illness is the result of functional body impairments which permit the accumulation of endogenously (internally) generated toxins. This condition is caused by enervation due to the exhaustive dissipation of the body's energies—and IS NOT an attack upon the body from the outside.

So long as the body's needs and supplies are met, no disease evolves. The human body is designed for efficiency and for high-level performance. To protect itself when threatened, it takes defensive measures in an effort to eradicate the threatening substance or influence.

The body will expend force and power beyond the norm to cleanse itself and to prevent a continual raid on its banked energy reserves. Only when functioning power has been reduced such that metabolic waste is incompletely expelled, nutrition impaired, secretion checked, and vital processes hampered, does the body become sick, embarking on an emergency course of restoration and liberation.

The body becomes sick because it strives to achieve the highest level of well-being possible. If loaded with toxins, it withdraws energy from normal channels and re-directs them to extraordinary purification processes to accomplish the expulsion of morbid material. If this did not take place, morbid material would collect until sufficiently concentrated to kill the organism.

The Organs of Detoxification and Their Role in Disease

The body organs most commonly involved in the processes of elimination, detoxification, purification, and cleansing are the lungs, kidneys, liver, colon or bowels, mucous membranes (internal skin), and the external skin.

As toxic material accumulates in the body and our normal channels of elimination become impaired or clogged due to exhaustion from abusive living, the body must have an outlet for waste material or we would soon perish. In seeking such an extraordinary outlet, the body uses all means available including acute fevers, colds, rashes, etc.

Acute symptoms (either mild or severe) represent an attempt by the body to cleanse itself of a burden too great for the system's normal eliminative channels to handle. These represent "safety valves" whereby the body creates an exudation point for wastes. Without a state of internal congestion due to intoxication, however, such disease symptoms would never be expressed.

The Remedial Effects of Acute Symptoms

Acute disease is a defensive action instigated by the body in an effort to correct a threatening situation to the organism. As such, it is a normal natural process of rectifying abnormal developments. Acute symptoms of fever, colds and flu represent the body's remedial process as it strives to maintain the status quo—homeostasis, or physiological equilibrium. Such action is always remedial.

These diseases are body instituted and conducted for the purpose of cleansing, repair, and restoration, and are self-limited to the amount of time and effort necessary to rid the organism of injurious substances. The most significant reason why acute disease manifests is our fundamental biological need for a pure body.

When the body reaches a state where retained wastes seriously impede normal vital functioning, the body organizes for a thorough cleansing and rejuvenating crisis. During the disease/healing process, the body marshalls its forces for remedial efforts by lowering or ceasing altogether immediately non-essential body operations.

The system then re-directs and concentrates the energy it has preempted to other more immediately vital operations—those of coping with the extraordinary task of detoxifying itself and repairing damaged tissues.

In a few days a massive ejection of waste is achieved—uncomfortable, but necessary and eminently worthwhile. Although the body does expend great reserves of energy during the healing crisis, it is a process of self-preservation.

Acute disease symptoms, then, include all the body's various efforts and expressions in expelling uneliminated wastes and toxic materials. When the body's circulation and tissues become clogged to the degree where the saturation reaches intolerable proportions, the body marshalls its resources for a radical eliminative crisis.

For example with the flu, the temperature rises, the head and nasal passages may become congested, coughing, sneezing and discharge of mucus may occur, and the appetite diminishes—all of which constitute cleansing efforts to unburden the body's vital organs.

Although these symptoms may not be as comfortable as medical treatments which occasion immediate relief, all of them ARE DESIRABLE and will run their course as the body rids itself of waste.

Acute disease does not attack the body, *but rather is produced by it* as a means of restoring health. Acute disease symptoms represent a positive physical response and are proof that the body is in the process of correcting whatever is wrong as waste material is forced from the body.

The body is very selective and ALWAYS aims for improvement and better health unless interference is too great.

Only then, do we fail to recover and further degenerate into chronic disease. The remedial nature of many acute disease conditions such as colds, fevers, swellings, inflammations, rashes, the flu, etc., furnish numerous examples of how the body always tends towards health unless we thwart the process.

Body activities mistakenly termed "disease symptoms" are actually modifications of similar physiological processes seen during health—fever, inflammation and diarrhea, for instance, are all exaggerated functions of body temperature, circulation, and bowel action whose purpose is to occasion rapid expulsion of toxic materials.

But keep in mind, *fever is caused by the same powers of life that produce normal body temperature; inflammation is caused by the same powers of life that cause normal circulation; and diarrhea is caused by the same powers of life that cause normal bowel action.* Defensive body actions such as fever and diarrhea, enable the body to eject and eliminate accumulated toxins that are harmful to the physiology.

Fever, for example, is a defensive measure initiated by the body—as temperature rises, more waste is burned, and accelerated circulation more quickly removes the toxic debris. In the infant, fever is often much more intensely vigorous than in the adult, whose healing power is relatively weaker from decades of physical abuse.

The body naturally becomes weak and listless during fever while it purges itself of poisons since energy is expended and rechanneled in the direction of detoxification, and withdrawn from the muscles and the extremities. The mind perceives physical weakness, but the physiology is actually becoming stronger as it purifies.

The fact that all available nervous and physical energies are redirected to the area that needs healing most, and that blood and nerve supply is withdrawn from the body's skeletal system and musculature, makes it natural to feel weak and listless. Ride it out however, as the body is in the process of recovery.

Inflammation is another healing response within the body. Whenever there is tissue damage as a result of injury, the damaged tissue cells produce histamines which cause tiny blood vessels to release fluid into the injured area.

Clotting occurs and nature literally builds a partition between the infected area and the rest of the body, whose effect is to prevent the infection from spreading. Body fluids cannot move outside the infected area and instead they build-up, causing the characteristic swelling of inflammation. This healing process should not be suppressed, otherwise even a mild infection could become fatal.

Nausea, vomiting, and diarrhea may also occur when a poison is ingested as the body dispels the substance as quickly as possible with the least harm to the system. When extremely putrefactive material in the digestive tract is potentially injurious to the rest of the body, the system may initiate either vomiting or diarrhea to quickly shunt it from the system.

Once in the stomach or intestine, this toxic material elicits feelings of discomfort and nausea until violent contraction ejects the waste. Sometimes this material is so morbid that the body will send it "upstream" where vomiting will only expose it to three to four feet of tubing (stomach, esophagus), as opposed to "downstream" where some 30 feet of tubing (intestines) will be exposed during diarrhea.

Following this, there is usually a feeling of relief and improved well-being. Diarrhea and vomiting are emergency body defensive mechanisms for preserving and protecting itself which should not be suppressed.

Even during disease, the body ALWAYS tries to restore and maintain normality. Abnormal body actions including nausea, vomiting, diarrhea, coughing, sneezing, frequent urination, skin eruptions, fever, pain, inflammation, expectoration, etc., are remedial struggles that represent the body's efforts to expel injurious substances and to recover a normal, healthy state.

Sinus problems, nasal drips, excess mucus, fevers, rashes, boils, pimples, blackheads and psoriasis are but extraordinary efforts of body cleansing—which would not be necessary if the body were relatively pure. These provide examples of how resistance and expulsion are self-preservative efforts on the part of the organism. The healthy vital body will reject anything that is irritating.

If vitality is lowered due to poor lifestyle patterns, it is difficult to expel certain toxins and the body may adopt another self-preservation technique—it temporarily stores them away in the body's fatty tissue, or within body generated sacs called cysts or tumors.

The body acts vigorously in protecting itself. It may erect hundreds of growths, cysts, boils, warts, pimples, tumors, etc. to quarantine internal hazardous substances and if necessary, it creates many extraordinary outlets as last resort measures to extend life and to save the organism.

The so-called "symptoms of disease," then, are just extensions and exaggerations of normal body activity that continue for as long as we provide the poisonous conditions that warrant their attention.

The Degenerative Effects of Chronic Disease

To reiterate, if diseases are remediable and reversible (as most of them are), it is *constructive*. When disease can no longer be reversed through body remediable processes, it is *degenerative* or chronic.

In cases of *acute* or reparative disease, symptoms are due to the active expulsion of toxins, but in cases of *chronic* degenerative disease, *the individual suffers symp-*

toms because of the injury the toxins have DONE to the system.

This injury usually occurs after constructive disease has been repeatedly checked, suppressed and interfered with over long periods of time by the administration of drugs, herbs, supplements or other therapeutic treatments and modalities. Many diseases commonly regarded as chronic can be corrected by the body however—most cases of arthritis being among them (provided the bones have not fused together during ankylosis).

Whenever any unwanted foreign material is ingested, all vital powers of the body that can be spared are employed in rendering the substance harmless. Defensive action by the body is *always* forthcoming—the extent to which it is established is wholly dependent upon the power which is available. The stronger and more vital, the stronger the response. The weaker and the more *chronically* toxic the individual, the weaker the response.

When causes are continued for any *prolonged* length of time, the acute healing crisis is transformed into chronic disease which the body conducts unceasingly. Organic tissue damage at this point has occurred from repeated violation of our body's needs, and can even bring about an end to life itself.

Illnesses said to kill thousands each year are not of themselves dangerous. Rather, the mortality seen in disease is due to suppressive and combative treatments.

Acute disease is not an enemy at war with the body. It is not something to be expelled, subdued, opposed, destroyed, conquered, cured, or killed, since it is not a "thing" or "an entity" at all. Rather, acute disease is an action, a process, a remedial effort to be cooperated with.

It is of utmost importance to understand that **the body resists the CAUSES of disease and NOT the disease itself.** Acute disease is used to eject toxins and maintain health.

As such, ***disease symptoms are a blessing in disguise.*** This reparative process should not be suppressed with drugs, otherwise chronic disease will develop. Relapses occur when medicinal substances are used for palliation and this is exactly what should be avoided.

The inherent healing power of the organism is the only force for restoring a salubrious state. Treatments interfere with self-healing, and should be avoided.

Any attempt to CURE disease by ADDING to its cause(s) is irrational and illogical. Hygienic care, on the contrary, involves the proper use of nature's materials and influences. An irreconcilable conflict exists, therefore, between "modern medicine" and the Hygienic system—if one is correct, the other is not.

The sick recover in accordance with the same laws of physiology which govern the body when in a state of health. Rarely does one *suddenly* get sick since physiological change of structure and function from health to disease is slow. Underminings often proceed for weeks, months, years and decades before disease becomes evident.

The essential condition of life is health—THIS IS THE NORM, AND DISEASE IS ABNORMAL. As surely as man is constituted to live, so is he constituted for health.

Hygienists do not recognize disorder in the vital domain—for in the biological realm, organic order reigns. Whether function is smooth as in health or uneasy as in acute disease, there is no lack of order.

Modifications of function such as fever, coughing, sneezing, inflammation, vomiting, diarrhea, etc., are not symptoms to be treated, cured, subdued, suppressed, or in any way interfered with. They develop in accord with physiological law only when there is a need for them, and persist only so long as the need persists.

Nearly all examples of abnormality called "disease" are due to habits and practices easily explained, and easily avoided. According to Natural Hygiene, diseases are symptomatic malfunctions that result from one or more of these detrimental factors:

1. Eating foods that we are not biologically adapted to;
2. Overeating; or eating excessively of foods in an unnatural state (cooked, processed, fragmented, refined or incorrectly combined in excess of our digestive enzyme capacity);
3. Ingesting toxic substances;
4. Taking drugs (prescription; over-the-counter; and/or recreational);
5. Insufficient sleep and rest;
6. Lack of fresh air;
7. Lack of vigorous exercise;
8. Lack of sunshine; and
9. Inability to cope with stressful situations.

According to Natural Hygiene, then, disease neither has to be fought nor prevented---if we meet our *simple* life requirements, illness will not occur. The *uncomplicated* task of maintaining health is all the disease prevention we need.

Natural Hygiene takes the opposite stance of today's modern sophisticated "disease" care system, that disease is natural and inevitable, and therefore needs to be fought off and prevented. Natural Hygiene, on the contrary, states that disease is NOT normal to the human organism except in abnormal circumstances.

Unhealthful Living and Increased Toleration to Toxins—Broken Down Resistance

As unhealthful living routines continue over the years, the body learns to tolerate more toxins and it develops fewer eliminative crises.

The constant introduction of poisons into the body either from external sources, or from the accumulated generation of metabolic waste products due to incorrect lifestyle habits, will damage cells, tissues, and organs as well as lead to an increase in the ***systemic toleration*** to toxins routinely encountered.

With increased toleration, the body constantly functions under a handicap, wasting vitality. As the body lives with more internal poisons, waste products remain to damage the system which then paves the way for future degenerative/chronic disease.

Toleration means that the body does not have sufficient vital energy to resist—toleration is submission, broken-down resistance. The body's self-protection has been gradually eroded. The organism is undermined and premature death is the final result.

The body pays for increased toleration by general enervation and lowered resistance to unhealthful influences. As resistance decreases, toleration increases as the body adapts to higher levels of internal toxicity. The system loses functioning power in the process and ages prematurely since its ability to ward off toxins diminishes.

The dictionary definition of tolerance is "the power or ability to endure, withstand or resist the effects of a drug or any physiological insult without showing unfavorable effects."

This definition is false, however, at least as far as health is concerned—for if the body endures any physiological insult,

IT IS BECAUSE OF A LACK OF STRENGTH TO RESIST. When the body does resist it is because it has the energy to institute defensive action: fever, diarrhea, vomiting, sneezing, or any crisis of cleansing and healing.

It is sad when the body tolerates poisons, for the repeated use of a poison (tobacco, alcohol, opium, heroin, cocaine, medical drugs and herbs, etc.) gradually overcomes and decreases the body's vitality.

When a cigarette is lit-up and inhaled for the first time, for example, the body responds with nausea, coughing, and dizziness as it tries to defend itself. If smoking continues everyday, however, the body raises its tolerance levels and accepts the toxic substances—the system becomes desensitized and weaker from this compromise. Symptoms disappear and addiction takes place.

The body is limited in the amount of vital resistance it can muster against the continued assault of intoxicating influences. Accommodation to smoking and other poisons imposes upon the body higher levels of toxicity, and the system also becomes disabled in its ability to normally excrete its own internally generated metabolic waste.

When tobacco, coffee, drugs, alcohol, etc., are consumed over the years, the body gradually loses its sensitivity and the result is impaired function and disease.

Those who eat all the wrong foods and get no exercise and seem to get along well have developed bodies with such a high tolerance level for morbid material that a weakening of the detoxifying organs has occurred. These individuals no longer have the vital strength to conduct necessary and effective eliminative crises, and toxins are dammed-up in the body.

Some people are blessed with superior genes and it takes a long time for their body to deteriorate into a irreversible degenerated condition—but improper living will eventually produce this outcome if the necessary "housecleaning" does not occur.

In the meantime, their way of life prepares the body for a long list of chronic diseases that grow out of established toxemia.

Adaptations, Accommodations, and Compromises in Health— Never Negotiate Your Well-Being

The body is extremely flexible—it will adapt to abnormal conditions, but such compromises will result in a lowered degree of health. The body adapts to whatever negative influences it cannot free itself of and tries everything possible to maintain functional poise in the midst of adversity, sacrificing well-being in the process. Functional vigor is lowered for the sake of survival. When the body is forced into compromise, it does so invariably at the expense of health.

Adaptation to poisons (the establishment of toleration) is accomplished by pathological changes in the body's tissues that are away from the ideal and which cripple normal function.

Adaptation to damaging influences, *even when successful* , is accomplished at great expense to the body as precious energy is wasted during its struggle to accommodate. When adaptation is UNSUCCESSFUL, the organism does not survive.

When the body's toxic level rises above a point of toleration, and poisons accumulate past a saturation or "tolerance" point, the body initiates a housecleaning and the organism takes remediable defensive and reparative action to protect itself.

When the body has established high toleration levels, acute disease does NOT eliminate *all* the toxins—it only lowers the toxic load to a level to which the body has become adapted. Colds and flu, for instance, are produced by body action to purify and cleanse the cells, tissues, and body fluids as made necessary by accumulations of toxic material beyond the body's ability to tolerate.

The body initiates a process of supplementary elimination where the mucus membrane of the nose and throat are requisitioned for vicarious duty in freeing the system of accumulated waste. The cold and flu does not eliminate ALL the toxemia, it only brings it down once again to a level at which the body has become adapted to functioning.

This adaptation is a compromise in order to preserve life; otherwise, the organism could not survive the tremendous energy expenditure and constant elimination required due to the ongoing incorrect modes of living and by decades of routine drug and medical treatments. Instead, the body adapts by sacrificing its potential for supreme health and vitality in order to survive. High toleration, however, CAN be returned to its pristine low level by fasting and then implementing a biologically correct lifestyle.

The toleration level of the average Hygienist, for example, has been reduced and his or her vitality restored to the point where his or her body no longer tolerates a large toxic load. Under this condition, the Hygienist's system may conduct extraordinary elimination at a much lower level compared to that which would allow *others* to continue insulting their bodies.

The stronger, purer body defends itself more rigorously against abuse in order to maintain its fitness, whereas the weaker the body, the more stimulation and attention it commands and the poorer it functions.

The body's ability to adapt to adverse circumstances is remarkable, but health is a delusion when we attempt to produce it with drugs. Under such conditions, the body will inevitably become exhausted, and chronic illness will ensue.

Chapter 10

THERE ARE NO CURES— OTHER THAN HEALTHFUL LIVING

Hygienic Health Care refutes present day notions that disease and ill-health are inevitable and that they depend on chance and circumstance beyond our control.

Instead, Hygiene states that health is obtained through healthful living—it cannot be bought over-the-counter at drugstores, found at the physicians office, nor within hospitals. Healing is entirely a biological process that unceasingly continues inside every organism unless this capacity has been debilitated with poisons.

Natural Hygiene does not believe in "cures"—rather, Hygienic practitioners assist the body in its self-healing by providing optimal conditions for healing to commence. This may entail a change in diet, a fast, a vigorous exercise program, stress management strategies, or combinations of these various lifestyle refinements.

The only source of healing is your own body. Hygienic Self-Health Care recognizes the living organism as dynamic and self-reparative so long as energy is abundant. This ability *always* functions in both sickness and health, as long as the system is not chronically enervated or debilitated.

There are no "cures" in medicine, in Hygiene, nor anywhere else since the true "cure" is nothing more than the correction of causes which necessitated disease in the first place.

The only way we can help this process is by providing ideal conditions for the body to implement its own self-healing capabilities. Such conditions are optimum during a fast, during which time healing is concentrated and multiplied—especially when followed by a biologically adapted dietary and lifestyle regime.

Natural Hygiene **DOES NOT** claim to cure disease, nor does it claim to reverse irreversible pathologies—it will not create new organs, nor prevent death when important organs are deranged and organically degenerated.

Hygiene, rather, makes full use of the life-sustaining means of nature, and places full reliance in *those* means that have a normal relation to human physiology. Life depends on organic harmony—where organic change is not TOO great, *permanently* removing the causes of functional derangement will allow the body to slowly regain normality.

What Hygienic care **DOES** claim is that where recovery is still possible by means of Hygienic materials and influences, health can be restored much more rapidly, safely, efficiently and more certainly than when these same essentials of health are neglected. As such, Hygiene solely depends upon the intrinsic, restorative forces of the body to perform the actual work of repair and reconstruction. **If this is quackery, then life itself is a quack and nature one grand cheat.**

As a matter of fact, **Hygienic Health Care is NOT involved in any way, shape, or form with curing illness** because all efforts to do so are based on false notions of the essential nature of disease—since acute illness IS the body's defensive/remedial process at work. Attempts to cure through medical substances prevents the body from performing its most basic healing functions.

In disease and health, then, we must supply the body with its primordial needs so it may continually build health—for this is the organisms natural tendency. ***This is why we do not have to MAKE the body healthy through curative agents; we only have to LIVE healthfully.***

What is necessary to produce life is also required for its preservation. The human body developed under certain natural conditions, influences, and materials that are essential to the maintenance of health. Those influences responsible for a human to grow into adulthood in a state of health and vigor, are all that is required to preserve that health throughout his or her lifetime.

Natural Hygiene is NOT a Therapeutic System of Healing

In Hygienic Health Care, the essentials of health—proper food, pure water, exercise, sunlight, rest, etc., are NOT employed as remedies; instead, the requisites of health *are* our normal requirements whether we are sick or well, and rest is the *condition* whereby the body restores its functional integrity.

Natural Hygiene is not a collection of therapies, nor is it

engaged in a ceaseless search after new, more novel, more sensational and miraculous cures. In the nearly 175 year history of Hygiene, *not one single cure has ever been brought forth by any Hygienic practitioner since there are no "curative agencies" in nature and as such, Hygiene recognizes none.* Disease is the result of physiological needs being violated, and only implementation of such needs provides true conditions of recovery.

Hygiene employs those means whereby health is sustained in order to restore it when lost. This system of health care is NOT a system of therapeutics; rather, it builds health in cases of disease through the employment of Hygienic agents *alone* , without the employment of drugs or palliatives of any kind. Constructive surgery forms the only non-hygienic measure endorsed by Natural Hygiene.

Hygienic Health Care does not claim that the body can overcome every obstacle, neither does Hygiene claim to *absolutely* avoid drugs or surgery in times of emergency first-aid, serious life-threatening accidents, or injury. The recommendation is, however, to avoid the causes of disease.

If medical intervention becomes necessary, conservative techniques should be used and every attempt made to support the body's inherent mechanisms for healing—for under normal conditions, when provided with the essentials of organic life and when stress is minimized, the physiology is completely self-regulating, self-directing, and self-healing.

In an article from the March/April 1993 issue of *Health Science* magazine entitled "Hygiene vs. Therapy," Ralph Cinque, D.C., describes how when people first utilize Natural Hygiene, they often have "clinical" goals to achieve—such as lowering blood pressure, normalizing weight, or overcoming disease, all of which serve to motivate them and to measure progress.

Self-Health Care, however, should NOT be thought of

in terms of therapy, therapeutic fasts, diets, exercises, etc., just because its results are often compared with the various therapeutic schools of healing.

When people implement Hygienic Health Care in their life and live in harmony with their body's legitimate needs as an alternative to therapeutic modalities, this does NOT mean that Natural Hygiene is itself a therapeutic system. Let's examine this further to see why this distinction is important to understand.

Hygienic Self-Health Care is comprised of specific lifestyle behaviors (and the avoidance of others) that satisfy our systemic needs while simultaneously preserving or restoring health to the greatest degree possible. Therapy, on the contrary, involves chemically or mechanically forcing the body to alter its structure or function.

While therapy involves FORCE, Hygiene involves modification of lifestyle BEHAVIOR towards alignment with our natural mandate. (Psychotherapy can be thought of in this perspective, as applying the force of ideas onto the patient's awareness). Forceful therapy is justified only when the body itself is unable to satisfy its organic needs through normal orderly physiological processes.

Circumstances such as a dislocated shoulder, setting a broken bone, an abscess that may require drainage, the removal of skin cancer, tumor obstruction that is not self-autolyzed, insulin deficiency in cases of irreversible diabetes, and so on, are just a few of the exceptions that in no way alter the essentials of health or establish normal standards of behavior.

To seek therapy in an emergency situation is one thing, but to add therapeutics to the lifestyle routine is counterproductive and outright dangerous—especially when therapy is not accompanied by education that teaches how to minimize it and how to regain health.

"Therapeutic Bias" and the Various Schools of Healing

Dr. Cinque also refers to the phenomenon of "therapeutic bias," that patrons of alternative therapists need to consider—the tendency of therapists to interpret health problems in such a way as to justify "need" for the particular therapy they offer.

For instance, allergists attribute headaches to allergies; but chiropractors attribute them to spinal fixations. Osteopaths blame headaches on cranial faults; nutritionists explore the possibility of nutritional deficiencies. Holistic dentists may advise that mercury amalgam fillings are causing the problem; an acupuncturist will locate a meridian blocking the flow of *chi.* Ayurvedic practitioners will proclaim your *doshas* out of balance and recommend *pancha-karma;* herbalists and homeopaths similarly would establish the need for their services. Finally, the allopathic physician would prescribe a painkiller and send you on your way.

Alternative therapies such as ayurvedic medicine, medicinal herbs, enemas, homeopathic remedies, acupuncture, spinal adjustments, crystals, visualization, etc., are popular as alternatives to traditional allopathic medicine solely because they appear to "work." Their prescribed modalities suppress symptoms of illness but often the underlying causes of disease remain intact—so the root of the problem remains.

There is always uncertainty involved with each of these therapies. They may make you feel better but they may also *cause* problems. The bottom line is that lifestyle practices or influences that caused the problem usually remain intact. Without education in the essentials of health, and corresponding adjustments in lifestyle behaviors, illness is likely to reappear sometime in the future.

While more popular schools of healing have largely confined their investigations to drugs, serums, surgical measures, high-tech equipment, manipulations, supplements, herbs, needles, magnets and crystals, these same schools commonly neglect or even belittle the potent essentials and means included under the banner of Hygiene.

While Hygiene strikes at the cause and corrects the conditions to which disease symptoms are due, the various "curing" systems involve themselves with the treatment of pain and palliation of discomforts, as if *these* where the enemies to be obliterated.

Instead, Hygienic Self-Health Care maximizes our quality of health and well-being because it is in harmony with our biological needs. Therapy, however, is inherently risky since it entails a departure from normal behavior, as well as breeding dependency rather than self-sufficiency.

Natural Hygiene studies health and its conditions, considering these to be the requirements of *restoring* a salubrious state and for *removing* the need for disease. In doing so, it seeks to remove those factors that impair the body. On the contrary, various schools of so-called "healing" all have their "cures" with which to combat disease—they find no need to supply the primordial requisites of well-being.

Because of all the conflicting claims made by the multitudes of healing modalities that are currently on the market, the decision whether to undergo therapy is often a difficult and confusing one.

The way to eliminate this confusion is to develop a permanent understanding of Hygienic Self-Health Care which enables you to accurately assess the body's genuine needs. In this way, the difference between healthful living and forceful intervention becomes clear and confusion is no longer an issue.

The function of Hygiene is to respect the laws of physiology. If we are to "aid nature" in times of disease, **we must**

know the nature of how our body operates and not interfere with life processes. Only when we possess such understanding can we intelligently cooperate with the natural self-healing forces of the body and cease throwing obstacles into our vital domain.

This knowledge allows for full confidence and reliance in Hygiene while simultaneously rejecting the myriad "cures" and "curing modalities" that exist in today's marketplace. The science of healing is the knowledge of the vital processes by which the living organism heals itself. When this science is widely acknowledged, Hygienic Self-Health Care will supplant "medical science" and many other "schools of healing."

A vast number of individuals who turn to Natural Hygiene in their search for health are very sick and do so as a court of last resort. Having attempted many different "healing modalities" that in the long run have failed, many finally arrive at Hygiene. Not all of these individuals can recover health, however, since Hygienic care relies on the vital forces of the organism—and these know no magic.

Often, when sick for prolonged periods of time, bodily structures slowly change—as tampering with drugs over years impairs the powers of life. Organs weaken, tissues are damaged, and circulation becomes sluggish. It takes years, if not decades, to arrive at such a ***dis-eased*** state and, as such, it is totally unreasonable to expect a few weeks or months of rest and fasting, plus a short time on a vastly improved diet to perform miracles.

Nature does not renew and refurbish a weakened, impaired state in short order. Just as there is no "magic bullet" via medical and alternative modalities, likewise, there is no miraculous way to health via Natural Hygiene.

SECTION IV

LET'S GET TECHNICAL:

THE "NUTS AND BOLTS" OF THE SELF HEALING BODY—WHY *SELF* HEALTH CARE WORKS

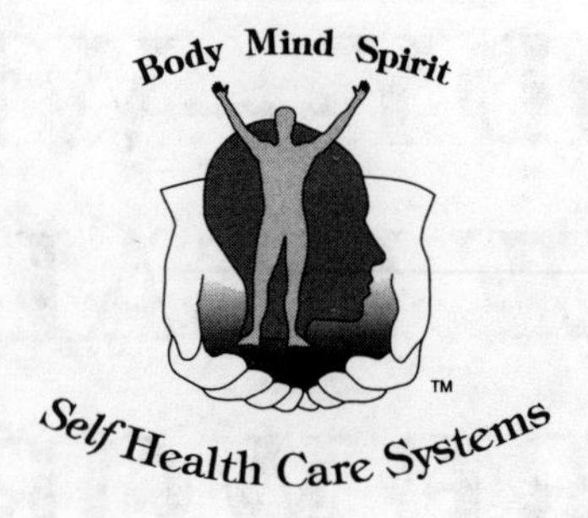
Body Mind Spirit
Self Health Care Systems

Chapter 11

THE BODY'S SELF-SUFFICIENCY AND UNITY OF FUNCTION: OUR PHYSIOLOGY "SELFISHLY" LOOKS AFTER ITS OWN WELFARE

The living body depends entirely upon the processes of nutrition and drainage (elimination) for its continuing existence. Nutrition and drainage, in turn, are dependent on the body's normal, efficient function—and normal efficient function, in its turn, is dependent upon our satisfactory attainment of the basic needs of life.

Foremost among the body's needs are fresh air, pure water, adequate rest and sleep, internal and external cleanliness, adequate sunshine, vigorous exercise, emotional poise, security of life, recreation and play, comfortable temperature, pleasant environment, constructive work, self-mastery, and perhaps most importantly, **FOODS WHICH WE ARE BIOLOGICALLY EQUIPPED TO UTILIZE.**

The ONLY things we should put into our body are distilled water, fresh air, sunlight, and a diet of mostly fresh, raw fruits supplemented with vegetables, nuts and seeds.

The body is self-sufficient so long as its needs are adequately met. It is a self-directing, self-defensive, self-purifying, self-repairing and self-healing organism. The body is also self-constructing from conception to maturity and beyond. In order to do its best under all circumstances, all the body requires is that its biological requisites be satisfied, and that it not be abused.

Life is shortened when deviation from our biological heritage occurs. The body becomes clogged and disabled by wrong foods and improper lifestyles that deplete our energy and vitality. Anything that impairs health also shortens life. The human body is hard to kill, but this is no reason to continue the abuse of our highly developed organism.

In spite of the stress and strain to which humankind is subject, however, the body is a self-balancing, self-preserving mechanism that promotes and maintains health to the best of its organic ability.

The human body has remarkable powers of self-regulation, adjustment, and distribution. When unhampered, the body distributes its available energy to its various organs and tissues in proportion to their requirements and importance.

The body is so much more serviceable, and performs so much better, when it is accorded the care it requires. If we live healthfully, the body might live to well over 100 years of age on *the average WITHOUT ANY ILL HEALTH OR SUFFERING.*

Body Structure and Function is a Wholeness, Greater Than the Sum of Its Parts

To understand how to live healthfully and how to avoid or overcome diseases, you must first conceive of the human body as one complete integrated unit and NOT a collection of individual parts. The structure and actions of a vital organism represent the expression of organic unity.

Our various *"physiological systems,"* including the "immune system," "nervous system," "digestive system," "circulatory system," etc., exist only as abstractions for purpose of intellectual study, but do not exist isolated in nature except as integral parts of a holistic organism. Each system in the body (and each organ and gland of each system) functions only for the whole and only by virtue that it belongs as a part of the whole.

In fact, the notion of distinct systems in the body is fiction. Physiology is so interrelated that the labelling of various body functions as distinct from the whole has little relation to actual systemic functioning. In both health and disease, there is a continuous unity of function throughout the body.

It is not difficult to realize that the various systems of the body exist as only abstractions. Take, for example, the "digestive system"—the mouth, stomach, and small intestine all are components of the body, but digestion and assimilation of foods could not occur without the brain and nerves of the "nervous system," nor without the hormone messenger molecules of the "endocrine system," nor without the smooth muscle of the "muscular system," or the connective tubing of the "circulatory system."

Every part of the human body is designed for a particular function in order to help preserve systemic integrity as a whole.

As such, the body should be thought of as a unified structure whose component organs, tissues, and cells work in harmony to maintain health and whose quality of life depends on the continuous cooperation and coordination of all its components. If one system is disturbed, the health and integrity of the entire organism is adversely affected.

Continued habits of living that waste the body's energy eventually result in inhibition of secretion and excretion—and consequent self-poisoning. Proper diet combined with all of the other aspects of a Hygienic lifestyle results in health for the entire body.

Likewise, however, all body functions are also systemically affected by a toxemic state when conditions of health are continually violated. The part of the body most laden with toxins is the first to react symptomatically but the effect is systemic as all organs and tissues suffer impairment.

We do not have a diseased organ or gland then, but a diseased body. If our kidneys or appendix are diseased, for instance, the rest of the body is as well. The kidneys or appendix serve as the focal point for the elimination effort, the exit point at which toxic matters are purged from the system. They become inflamed with toxins because THE BODY is overloaded.

Body intelligence distributes this poisonous overload throughout all of our eliminative channels but despite this, the load is SO great that the kidneys or appendix become overburdened with more than they can handle. This condition is the same in all remedial disease where a local organ seems to be the only body part affected.

Even though disease affects the entire body, it also serves an important purpose—body detoxification. The body creates the disease/healing crisis in response to a physiological need to free itself of toxic material and repair damaged tissue.

A cold, for example, is not a cleansing of the "respiratory system" or of our mucus membranes but is an effort of systemic body purification. Likewise, hepatitis is not a "disease of the liver," rather, it is a total body-instituted effort at cleansing in which the liver is inflamed. *The entire body is toxic,* the liver is NOT the only diseased part. The same is true down the line for all diseases---all are the result of TOTAL body toxicity and represent systemic cleansing efforts that benefit the entire organism.

Understanding the UNITY of the functioning body is critical in understanding the body's actions in both health and disease. Unfortunately, we are taught to think of the body as a collection of systems, organs, glands, and separate (although interconnected) parts.

This conception of the human organism is erroneous and it leads to further misconceptions including the false idea that certain drugs, herbs, and foods "cleanse" or "heal" isolated organs without affecting the whole—when in fact, the body always reacts systemically to everything introduced therein.

To "treat" individual symptoms and isolated parts of the body is to ignore the very purpose of the body. This unbalanced approach thwarts the body's efforts and forces upon it an inimical condition it was striving to cast off. Even though it is convenient to study *parts* of the body and for medicine to treat isolated organs and affected diseased parts, the body's wholeness is ALWAYS greater than the sum of its component parts.

When we understand how the body operates in both health and disease, then we know how to cooperate with its efforts at self-healing and self-preservation. Only when we are aware of the dynamic, active nature of the human organism are we able to understand disease processes and how to attain and maintain health—for these are automatic processes, so long as we supply the basic needs of life.

There are just two categories of substances that enter or occasion contact with the body: those that afford nourishment (food); and those that have no normal relationship to the human body. If a substance bears no normal relation to the body, and if it is not generally used in any of its biochemical or physiological processes, then it does not belong in the body at all.

The only authority we should rely on when it comes to determining what food is best to eat, is the body. Physiology and anatomy is what makes food "acceptable" or "harmful" in the diet. Food consists of those substances which are useful in building protoplasm, cells, tissues, and organs; in healing and repair; and as a source of sufficient energy for performing metabolic functions and for fuel to maintain body temperature.

The processes of nutrition include the physiological processing the body conducts as it transforms food into material for its own growth and maintenance. A living organism at the cellular level grows, multiplies and reproduces itself and by this repetition, extends its life. To do this, the body's cells select from their environment suitable materials to transform into its own structure, while simultaneously rejecting and refusing all other substances. These physiological conditions are necessary to maintain the system's integrity.

Always, it is the BODY That Acts on Ingested Substances, Rather Than the Materials Acting on the Body

From a purely physiological standpoint, nutrition can be described by the mechanical and chemical actions of the body upon ingested foodstuffs. THE BODY IS THE **ACTIVE** AGENT AND FOOD IS **PASSIVE**—THE **BODY** ACTS UPON FOOD, FOOD DOES NOT ACT UPON THE BODY.

Food is inert and has no power to create living

tissue. Food cannot act but rather, *is acted upon* as the living body uses what it can of the consumed food's nutrients and rejects the rest.

The body acts in an orderly and purposeful manner in all its actions as it maintains and repairs itself in response to modifications in its environment. The human body is not a passive entity, rather it acts dynamically and intelligently on all substances introduced within.

Digestion is always entirely under control of the body. **Specific foods CANNOT "aid" digestion anymore then they can aid *breathing!*** UNSUITABLE foods can disrupt digestion through their toxic nature, but food itself is inert—it can do nothing. Food cannot perform active organic processes to build cells and tissue, but rather provide the raw materials for such action.

As such, there are no "healing foods," for when eaten, foods do nothing—it is the body that acts upon them. Food is either digested and assimilated or eliminated. **It is a mistake to consider that anything eaten goes into the body with intelligence, purpose, and an ability to locate our stored filth and physiological impairments in order to cleanse us and to create or repair our cells and tissues. ONLY THE BODY HAS THIS CAPACITY.**

The notion that foods have no power to act upon the body distinguishes Natural Hygiene from more traditional schools of nutrition. The idea of "food therapy," that certain foods perform specific actions in the body to effect a treatment or cure, *is false* . There are no "cures" whether they be in the form of foods, juices, medicines or herbs—the body is a self-healing organism and functions as such so long as its biological requirements are continuously met.

Once again, food is material for use by the body. *FOOD DOES NOT **DO** ANYTHING* —for it is done unto BY the body (that is, digested, absorbed and metabolized). **The primary**

requisite for better health is the removal and avoidance of foods and substances NOT suited to our constitution.

Just as the finest foods, influences, and lifestyle practices provide the best raw materials for the body in *building and maintaining life* on the highest possible level, so does faulty lifestyle, second-rate "non-foods," and energy-sapping influences *lower our well-being, and impair and destroy life* long before its time.

Most individuals use and unconsciously abuse their bodies carelessly, often believing that the body is made to function no matter what they do. While often overstressing their system and putting into it whatever food will satisfy "hunger" and "tastes good," when they do not feel well they regularly blame it on old age or "the bug that's going around"—but NEVER on their own self-abuse.

Gradually when their system breaks down, they search for relief with drugs without realizing that they have to change their lifestyle. Instead, they believe they will somehow be miraculously healed. After all, why do for YOURSELF what a few pills will do for you instead?

Chapter 12

THE HARM OF ALLOPATHIC (WESTERN) MEDICINE—THE ILLUSIONARY "ACTION" OF DRUGS AND SUPPLEMENTS

Any substance that is not adapted to the body's normal metabolic processes cannot be of use in conditions of either health or disease—such substances must be expelled. Those substances that are non-usable in a state of health are equally non-usable in a state of ILL-health.

Poisons are those influences that are chemically dangerous or those that are relatively inert but offer no nourishment. If the substance cannot be metabolized and employed into the body's normal nutritive processes, it is useless and treated as a poison.

If it possesses a strong chemical affinity for any cellular constituents, the tendency of the two to unite must be resisted. If the substance is not a normal constituent of the body's tissues, the work of expelling it is often painful and very costly to the body's economy.

When nonusable substances are brought into contact with the cells, the body resists, rejects, and expels them. All substances introduced into the body either by injection, absorption, respiration, or by ingestion which cannot be utilized as food by the organism are poisonous. Poisons are always acted upon by the body in self-defense.

DRUGS ONLY ACT CHEMICALLY AND ONLY CAUSE DAMAGE TO THE BODY. When two chemical substances unite, the resulting compound differs from the former substances. Tissue constituents and body cells die in the process, as the body's resistive, defensive, and expulsive actions are employed to prevent the chemical union from furthering damage to the system.

These actions have long been mistaken for actions of the poisons but actually, these activities are the living organism's attempt to cast off materials that cannot be normally appropriated into living structure.

Because of the body's self-preservative instincts, substances introduced into the organic domain that it cannot use are resisted by the entire organism. When the body is stimulated with drugs and/or medicinal herbs, the stimulating effect is the BODY'S RESPONSE to an unwanted agent and represents the body's efforts to eliminate it as quickly as possible by speeding up the circulatory system.

The body acts as a whole to expel the drug before it damages any one part too greatly by accelerating its metabolism such that the harmful substance will be quickly eliminated.

When drugs are taken, the first thing the body does is attempt to organize its resources for the drugs removal through the bowels, kidneys, liver, lungs, skin, the mucus membranes, by vomiting, etc. Noxious materials are either rejected or, if this for later expulsion.

Cells, tissues, and organs are damaged in resisting and expelling drugs, which causes impaired function. If organic tissue damage occurs due to repeated poisoning over extended periods of time, complete recovery may be impossible as chronic, degenerative disease sets in.

Drugs appear to "act" on particular areas of the body depending upon the particular drug's chemical composition. The emetic drug combines chemically with the stomachs constituents and causes damage; the purgative combines chemically with the bowels and causes irritation; aspirin (salicyclic acid) erodes the stomach wall and abnormally accelerates the heart as the body seeks to remove the aspirin before injury occurs.

Likewise, purging prevents further damage to the bowels from the chemical union between the drug and the organ's constituents. Likewise with vomiting, which EXPELS the poison before it chemically combines with tissues of the stomach.

Remember, when we take drugs the ensuing reactions such as sedation, palpitation, sweating, stimulation, diarrhea, vomiting, etc., ARE ACTIONS OF THE BODY. These are defensive, remedial and eliminative actions on behalf of the organism defending itself against the poison.

THE BODY ACTS ON THE DRUG ACCORDING TO THE DRUG'S CHEMICAL CHARACTER, using the point of least resistance for counter-active and eliminative measures which pose the least ill effects.

The protective efforts of the body AGAINST medi-

cine is misinterpreted as the beneficial actions of drugs. These reactions are said to be beneficial as the poison "causes the body to clean itself out." What is actually taking place, however, is that the body is resisting the toxin and making a heroic effort to eject and expel the substance. This DOES NOT represent a "curing crisis" brought on by the medicine.

When topical medicine and herbs are applied to external wounds (including aloe vera, comfrey, etc.) the outside of the abrasion closes faster than it normally would—this defensive response protects the body from irritating foreign matter (aloin, etc.) so that it is not absorbed into the system. As a result, proper healing may be interfered with and impaired.

The living body reacts to everything within its environment—to assimilate useful nutritional agents and influences and eject nonusable and destructive substances. *These two factors, the quantity and destructiveness of the toxic agent or influence and the vital energy of the organism, determine how the body reacts in every situation to what it encounters.*

The continuence of life depends upon the body's ability to channel any toxic overload to various accessory exit points whenever a life-threatening emergency situation presents itself.

Once again, the force mistakenly attributed to "medicinal action" is in actuality the VITAL POWER OF THE BODY. Medicines do not act at all, do not furnish power for action, and do not somehow impart power to the body for ITS own action. The action occurring between the body and drugs is exclusively vital action—POWER BEING EXPENDED, NOT GENERATED.

And because the living organism has performed all the action, its energy is depleted in proportion to the work it did to eliminate the poison. Functioning power is lowered and rest is needed to recover as the body is now in a weakened state.

When drugs are taken regularly over an extended period,

it is mistakenly believed that they gradually lose there effect—larger doses are then administered since the drug no longer has the ability to "act" effectively. What actually occurs, however, is that the drug NEVER had any power to act—instead, as a result of continuous expulsive efforts made by the body, our physiology loses ITS power to produce the same vigorous action and becomes weaker from the constant exhaustion.

Debilitated elderly people, for instance, cannot resist drugs as well as healthy youngsters since body vitality wanes over the years from the accumulative effects of improper living. The natural resistance of the body is lowered progressively due to violation of the laws of health, and the body compensates by not reacting as violently as when it was vital and vigorous—its defensive powers are slowly reduced.

The debilitated person, then, has less energy to expend in eliminating the drug. ***If the drug truly acted, it should act with MORE force in a weak person because of less resistance from weak organs—but we see just the opposite.***

Consider for a moment that if you introduce a drug into a dead body there is no action, whereas if the drug DID perform action, there should be MORE activity because there would be less resistance from the dead person's tissues than from living tissues.

But the obvious fact is that the dead body cannot vomit the drug, it cannot develop diarrhea, nor do its kidneys function to expel it. The drug does nothing except chemically combine with the constituents of the dead body's tissues.

And this is the difference between drugging a living body and a dead body—the live person resists the chemical union. As long as it is alive it will continue to do so since if allowed to proceed unchecked the chemical combination with cellular constituents would mean death of the cell. The living body fights to prevent this chemical union and in doing so, sometimes dies in the struggle. Cellular life has to die first before drugs can completely combine with cellular constituents.

Drugs can never have any "remedial" or "restorative action" for they possess no intelligence whatsoever. Drugs are not selective in their action for they have no discriminative ability with which to govern selection—instead, blind undirected chemical action is their only capacity.

All such action is detrimental to the living organism and in the process, much harm is done by interfering with normal life processes. The so-called "active properties" of medicine are actually MORBIFIC EFFECTS.

Drugs only derange body homeostasis and interfere with its operations. Drugs cannot clean the body out, rather they pollute it and destroy cells and tissues. If medicines where healthful we would live from pharmacies, not gardens and orchards.

The natural healing power of the body is behind all "cures" whether under the auspices of "natural therapies" including herbs, manipulations, acupuncture, hydrotherapy, electrotherapy, mineral and vitamin therapies, etc., or *in spite of* these medically oriented therapies.

Even when taken in small quantities , all drugs and "medicinal herbs" are poisons and always do harm. Homeopaths prescribe drugs in such minute doses that the body can eliminate these poisons much more readily than the large doses regularly prescribed by the medical doctor.

The body, therefore, is relatively unhampered in its healing efforts, **and it is the body that heals and effects the "cure"—not any drug.** Homeopaths would even be more successful if they prescribed NO drugs at all and addressed themselves to removal of causes.

Allopathy is a type of medicine that relies heavily on surgical procedures and the use of medications, and whose practitioners receive training from a recognized academic school of medicine.

Allopathy literally means "opposite disease." In theory, allopaths strive to displace the original disease by creating a heteropathic or opposite disease. Actually, all that physicians succeed in doing is creating ADDITIONAL disease in the body.

Allopathy is a system of medicinal practice involving the use of drugs which produce effects DIFFERENT from those of the disease treated. Allopathy DOES NOT aim at determining nor removing the *cause* of illness but, rather, the palliation of symptoms through a "magic bullet" approach which totally disregards the intelligent healing abilities of the body.

By treating symptoms, allopathic physicians are really not dealing with the disease at all—since the disease DOES NOT exist as an entity in and of itself but, rather, is created by the body as the means of purging itself of accumulated internal toxic waste.

By treating only symptoms which ARE evidence of body purification, the disease/healing process is halted to the detriment of the organism. Poisons are not only dammed up within the body, but the addition of "medicinal" drugs further poisons the physiology.

Medicines Create Iatrogenic Disease

Allopathy means to create a parallel affliction to overcome another affliction—to cure disease by creating another disease by using "remedies" whose "actions" are opposed to the symptoms caused by the disease entity blamed.

The allopathic school of modern medicine has actually brought new plagues into being, so-called iatrogenic diseases—illnesses caused by drug treatment intervention. Drugging stops the body's natural healing efforts and further poisons the system. NO drugging procedure can ever possibly remove the causes of disease. Palliation is an illusionary "cure," which actually leads one closer to death.

It is the tradition of allopathic medicine that the strongest poison is the best defense against disease. When it is falsely believed that disease is something that attacks you, the responsibility for one's health is then removed from the patient and put into the hands of "professional" doctors who practice poisoning to "cure" disease.

In Natural Hygiene, there is no attack since there is nothing to be attacked. The notion of "attack" apparently originated with ancient shamanism and voodoo religions who believed in "attacking entities" in the form of evil spirits. Viruses, germs, and bacteria have replaced these entities but are treated virtually the same.

Allopathy is primarily concerned with providing relief from symptoms rather than removing the underlying cause and provides little or no knowledge of how to create health—the system has nothing to do with healthful living. It stifles the body's natural healing efforts, whose symptoms are misunderstood as malevolent disease entities which must be killed off with the arsenal of allopathic drugs.

Any allopathic modality involving drugs, therapies, treatments, manipulations, herbs, etc., are infringements on the vital domain and cannot possibly assist the body in any way. On the contrary, they actually interfere with natural body detoxification efforts and normal reparative functions.

Such interference poses additional problems for the body to cope with and further lowers body vitality. In fact, vitality is lowered so much by the danger presented by allopathic drugs and/or other modalities (including herbs) that the original disease/healing effort is discontinued in favor of devoting available energies to the more virulent enemy and danger at hand—the administered drugs.

The original disease problem remains when allopathic drugs are employed but the body must re-direct its energies partly or wholly to removing the more dangerous so-called "medicines." The symptoms of the original disease disappear because the necessary energy and vitality to further conduct the disease/healing process is now lacking.

Yet the body is in graver danger than before it was "medicated," both from the uneliminated toxic accumulations and the added toxicity of drugs or other substances administered.

Instead of being helped, the body is placed in double jeopardy when using allopathic modalities. When drugs are administered to sick people, the same thing occurs as when they are administered to healthy people—TOXEMIA IS INCREASED, NOT DECREASED. The body must then expend energy to expel the drug rather than continue to eject internal toxins which generated the symptoms in the first place.

This is why symptoms disappear during drug administration—*because healing ENDS and the body redirects its energies in order to handle the toxic drugs which present more of an immediate emergency to the body's survival.*

How Medicines "Work"

Drugs "work" only in the sense that they occasion a slowing or stopping of the body's purification efforts in two ways: *first,* the body diverts its eliminative efforts to the expulsion of the drug since its immediate threat to the survival of the organism is greater than the stored toxins; and *second,* drugs, over time, so poison the body that it is unable to muster the vitality required to eliminate accumulated toxic saturation within the system.

As mentioned earlier, acute illnesses are body processes whose purpose is to set a wrong internal situation right. The crisis is carried on by the body in order to eliminate harmful toxins and to correct imbalances. No "cures," therefore, should be sought—the body should be left alone and allowed to carry out its cleansing process WITHOUT INTERFERENCE.

In all types of acute illness the entire body is occupied in the task of eliminating toxins as indicated by symptoms including mucus excretion, nausea, vomiting, fever, diarrhea, coated tongue, bad breath, anorexia, etc. The body at this time is unable to digest food since digestive power has been diminished and re-channeled to the eliminative tasks at hand.

To feed during the healing crisis only adds to the body's toxic load since food may readily ferment and/or putrefy. *WITHOUT* the irritating presence of food and its products of decomposition, the body will proceed to heal and health will be restored.

Do not interfere with or abort this self-healing process by adding anything to the body except pure (distilled) water. Even the best available foods are potential poisons during acute illness.

Likewise, using treatments, drugs and herbs, or anything abnormal and unnatural to the body interferes with healthful body functions and under no circumstances do such agencies improve or help the system.

To mistake disease action as an attack by an invader that must be routed with drugs is disastrous in practice. Much suffering results from the idea that the body is aided by outside "healing substances." Instead, these devitalizing agents depress body purification actions and reparative functions and suppress symptoms which are actual evidence of the body's healing efforts.

Because the body discontinues vital action required to purge the system of internal toxins and, instead, turns its energies towards removing the newly ingested poisons symptoms of the reparative process disappear—and the anti-vital effects of drugs and treatments are mistaken for healing effects.

Even more harmful, dangerous, and more difficult to

eliminate than various systemic poisons that originate within the body, are the medicinal drugs and serum injections administered to "cure" disease.

Medical and herbal "cures" decrease the body's strength and vitality. Herbs present less of an obstacle to the body, however, than the harsh concentrated drugs administered during medical treatment. Nevertheless, herbs and drugs destroy—they never build protoplasm. Drugs or herbs cannot create cells and replace body tissue. Drugs do nothing more than form destructive chemical unions with the body's compounds and fluids, and the body then suffers distress.

Any alien substance introduced into the body interferes with body functions, destroying or pathologically modifying them. ***Drugs and herbs "work" by occasioning the body to speedily expel them. This vital eliminative action by the body is mistakenly cited as "proof" that drugs are active "curing agents."***

Drugs work in much the same way as a lazy housekeeper sweeps dust under the rug—drugs cover up symptoms but do not remove the cause of disease. Our body is like the rug in that it only allows the drug to cover up the problem for so long.

Eventually, acute disorders become chronic, resulting in a more difficult condition for the body to deal with unless the causes are removed and one's lifestyle changed to one more in line with our biological needs.

By promoting "cures," medicine and herbology do nothing to remove the true causes of disease. People think that by swallowing a pill or plant they can improve their health, but the use of any curing agent only perpetuates the ignorance that enslaves people. *Health is only generated through healthy livng.*

At best, drugs and herbs temporarily give the ILLUSION of health and the person is WORSE off since they are not inclined to institute correct and healthful lifestyle practices.

The body, instead, continues to degenerate. By administering herbs or drugs, one endeavors to provide the diseased body with greater means of carrying on its healing efforts. Poisonous drugs are used in sickness because there is an effort to kill something—germs, parasites, or "viruses."

Although this war is nominally waged on disease, the warfare actually devolves upon the human constitution. *By sending into the body or applying to it, exotic toxins that cannot be used even in a state of health, the body is actually FURTHER debilitated.* The futile effort to cure disease in this fashion merely produces ADDITIONAL disease.

Medicinal Substances Suppress Symptoms of Self-Healing

When drugs are ingested, the body marshalls its available sources to handle the abnormal threatening substance. During this time, the organism HALTS reparative/healing processes which are felt as symptoms—thus, temporary relief. As soon as the foreign substance is disposed of, however, the body reinstitutes the healing process and old symptoms return, provided there is sufficient vitality.

Each time the body makes progress in its work, it receives a shock with the dispensing of drugs which suppresses detoxification efforts and decreases the body's vitality. Acute-/constructive disease **IS** evidence of body vitality, however, and drug treatment and medical therapy is therefore antivital—destructive of the body's faculties.

It is unwise to suppress disease symptoms because this stifles the body's attempt to heal. Symptoms of the disease-/healing crisis should not be suppressed but instead, left alone to complete their task. All curative properties reside solely within the human organism—no outside "healing agent" can simulate, stimulate, or motivate any inherent healing capabilities of the body.

The goal of every cell is to maintain life but drugs poison cells, and the body itself is killed off to some degree. In this way, drugs throw obstacles in the path of cells in their effort to support our well-being.

Rather than sabotage the body, assist life by providing the best conditions for health. **If substances are harmful to the body in health, they are also harmful in disease. Medical "science" is strange in that it advocates taking substances which make us sick when we are well in order to "cure" us when we are "stricken."**

Drugs and herbs do not have the property to act specifically upon the body—but the body does respond to anything which enters it. No drug or toxin of any kind has an effect on a single isolated tissue or organ. The body's circulation flows freely to every unit of life within and the effects of any drug or irritant are wholly systemic.

When drugs or herbs are particularly toxic, or taken in large doses, or if the individual is particularly weak and of low vitality, the result of administering the medicine may be almost complete cessation of the disease/healing effort—the body may be temporarily incapable of purging itself of accumulated filth as well as the poison in the drug or herb. The body then shows no or few symptoms of disease but is, in fact, MORE diseased and more toxic than before.

To repeat, *taking medication is merely symptom masking—the symptom of a diseased or disordered body is hidden by the body's eliminative efforts to rid itself of the medical substance.*

As such, medical treatment is suppressive and NEVER removes cause. Rather, it lowers the body's functioning power, impedes the body's healing efforts of self-detoxification, and causes the retention and greater toleration of more and more toxic matter.

Our susceptibility and vulnerability to future chronic disease is then increased.

It normally takes years of body mismanagement and multiple physiological errors to produce the pathological process of cancer. Drugging suppresses symptoms, and the disease process once again must be stimulated at a later date to detoxify and heal the body.

In the meantime, cellular growth becomes progressively deranged as drugs continue to sequester symptoms. Toxicosis continues, as does the evolution of disease, which expresses itself years later, often in horrendous ways. Sooner or later, the body will face an ever increasing serious situation—perhaps pneumonia, bronchitis, hepatitis, cancer, or AIDS.

Symptoms may be suppressed with drugs and the illusion of a "cure" may appear but such "recoveries" never truly result in a state of health. Suppression of one symptom results in a worsened condition that may eventually reappear in the same location or elsewhere.

Symptoms should not be suppressed or interfered with, but should be cooperated with. *Do not try to "cure" this healing process* —the body is healthier as it throws off more and more wastes that eventually would bring on serious disease, pain, and prolonged suffering and premature death. When symptoms are present, the more rest and sleep taken, the more quickly healing progresses and symptoms disappear.

We should seek to supply Hygienic conditions and materials which the laboring body can make constructive use of, including fresh air, pure water, sunshine, adequate rest and sleep, exercise and emotional poise. The body may then carry forward its restoration to a successful completion.

When the body is diseased, only those substances and influences that are NOT foreign but usable and necessary factors in a state of health should be supplied. Only they can be of any advantage to

us. When sick, therefore, the body is NOT able to appropriate substances that would contribute to ill health if taken under normal conditions.

The body is not an opponent to be battled against with drugs but is an intelligent, immeasurably complex living system that automatically will seek its own highest welfare when allowed to do so. Given favorable conditions, the body will spontaneously heal itself.

Just because we do not understand the body's functioning does not give us licence to assault it with drugs, serums, or unnecessary supplementation. To do so may only lead to permanent injury.

Stimulants and Supplements, Literally a Waste of Energy—Whipping the Body Out of Shape

The body's physiological reaction to medicine, herbs, and supplements is the creation of a stimulating effect within certain organs to remove the poisonous substances. The kidneys, liver, and lungs are commonly called upon to dispose of toxic drugs which eventually abuses, overworks, and impairs these organs.

If nutrient overload from dietary supplementation takes place which cannot be stored or disposed of immediately, the body will temporarily "dump" it somewhere in the system where it interferes as little as possible with normal systemic function and still be tolerated. The body then instigates measures to remove it as fast as possible when opportunity permits.

To accomplish the "dumping" or the rapid exodus of any foreign or excess substance, the body is stimulated by the nervous system to dramatically increase its metabolic action. Stimulation produces a false "high," and, for this reason, the nutritional supplement or stimulant appears to make the person feel better.

This false exhilaration may become habit forming, as in caffeine, but only too soon does the body become accustomed to the stimulating presence and, when deprived of it, goes into withdrawal and sinks to an unexpected lower level of depression.

Stimulation, then, is a forced draft upon the energies of the body. It compels energy EXPENDITURE, not by doing useful work but by resisting the stimulant. The depletion of the body's energy is commensurate with the amount of stimulation it is subjected to.

Stimulants which threaten cellular integrity by abnormally revving-up body metabolism must always be differentiated from the stimulation and revitalization which are observed following proper nutrition which serves to renew body reserves—referred to as COMPENSATORY STIMULATION.

Any stimulant which is *uncompensated* brings about the expenditure of the body's vital power which stimulants do not and cannot supply. Once the power is used, it is depleted and lost. This is why exhilaration induced by drugs and other stimulants is always followed by weakness. With the constant use of uncompensated stimulants, the strength and vitality of the body is gradually tapped and drained away.

We seem stronger in the short term when we use drugs, herbs and commercial vitamins and mineral supplements only by the expenditure of our vital force—but we grow weaker as they steadily draw upon the body's reserve energy supply.

Today's medical practice continually pumps the weak person with drugs and/or supplements to goad them into a false sense of well-being. But efforts to stimulate, sustain, invigorate and "kick-start" the tired, sick body always produces an equal and opposite reaction—depression of vigor and function.

One of the foremost characteristics of poisons is that they

stimulate, or goad the body into a frenzy—actually, the body steps-up energy EXPEDITURE to cope with a heavy eliminative situation. Because this makes us feel "hyper," we are likely to mistake this squandering of energy as being derived from the toxic substance ingested rather than a draft on our energy stores.

Nutritional supplements often provide a strong stimulus to the body just as does any toxin or foreign agent. This stimulus is often mistaken for a beneficial effect but is actually the body's response to an unnatural and inorganic presence—especially when ingested in the large quantities commonly suggested. On the other hand, the nutrients that naturally occur in whole foods are present in the correct synergistic proportions as needed by the body.

Drugs, nutritional supplements, vitamin and mineral pills, coffee, tea, nicotine, alcohol, herbs, onions and garlic all do lasting harm by reaching into the body's energy reserves to accomplish the "good" they appear to do while offering nothing in return of lasting value. Their efforts and affects are cumulative and remain with the person who employs them.

Remember, the body derives its energies from CARBOHYDRATES, not vitamins, minerals, supplements, drugs, junk foods or anything else. Euphoria occasioned by their use is ALWAYS followed by depressed functioning due to the expenditure of power required to bring about the exhilaration in the first place.

This fact is born out *most* clearly when those who partake heavily of nutritional supplements, vitamin or mineral pills, herbs or garlic concoctions, etc., decide to kick the habit cold turkey. The common experience is a series of withdrawal symptoms, usually involving depression, nervousness, irritability, and the "heebie-geebies"—all of which continue until the body purges itself of the offending stimulants.

Anything which abnormally causes the body to increase its metabolic action is a stimulant. The body "sounds an alarm" in times of danger and immediately accelerates body action. This effect is a defense mechanism to insure immediate survival whenever any toxic or irritating substance or influence is introduced into the body. All increased action occasions extra energy expenditure in order to cope with undue stress of any kind.

We are only conscious of the body's lack of energy after its reserves have been raided too often, when our power supply is low. Vitality or energy is usually noticed only in its expenditure, rarely in its accumulation. Like our car battery we only see its energy at work but we are unable to see its energy stored within.

Similarly, during sleep we display no sign of regeneration taking place in the slumbering body. Whereas rest and sleep restore our energy depleted reserves, and sound nutrition also replaces reserves that are expended during metabolism, stimulants cause power to be drained and do not replace the power which is expended.

The power of the body to generate energy is limited; the power of the SICK body to generate energy is crippled. The sick person suffers from nervous fatigue and exhaustion as a result of a previous waste of energy. Drugs, supplements, treatments, or any measure that further depletes energy stores do not help. Instead, these abnormally stimulate the body which wastes more energy and, like whipping a tired horse, the body becomes further enervated.

All stimulants, therefore, are useless to the system. They cannot be turned into cellular substance, tissue, blood, or protoplasm. Stimulants represent an encumbrance to the body, a threat to its efficiency and a hindrance to its normal, healthy function.

Stimulants, unfortunately, do much *more* harm than merely causing the body to accelerate the speed of vital organs, tissues and cells and do more than waste the body's vital energy reserves. More importantly, stimulants inflict injury upon the cells and tissues with which they come in contact. Cells harden to protect themselves from further injury as skin develops callouses from repeated irritation.

Because of their wounding, cellular functional capacities are compromised and diminished. Stimulants, and megadoses of nutritional herbs, and supplements (like drugs) suppress but never solve the problem of ill health. On the contrary, they add to the problem itself by further weakening our organs.

Aspirin, antihistamines, antibiotics, and ALL drugs stop the body from performing its intended purification tasks. This dams-up the poisons and multiplies the body's problems. Even so-called "natural cures" including herbs, vitamin C supplements, etc., thwart the body's actions with similar potential damage to physiological processes.

Taking supplements whether vitamins, minerals, amino acids, protein powders, etc., is anti-health in nature. ANY nutrient taken in excess of the body's needs become toxic and either must be removed from the system or stored, which may result in a toxic overload.

To the extent that the body diverts energy to the expulsion of drugs, herbs, or supplements to that extent a reduction in vital action occurs elsewhere in the body. The usual result is a reduction in the remedial/healing process—*not by removing its causes but by a reduction of the body's vital power which conducts the disease process itself.* Such a reduction comprises suppression.

Drugs and supplements literally flood the system with concentrations of abnormal substances and occasion defensive action. The difference between a diet predominating in fresh fruits and vegetables and a deficient diet is that fruits are food the body can use in a physiologic manner, whereas deficient diets and supplements introduce conditions in which the body expends its resources for purposes of protection and extraordinary excretion.

The human body can utilize only a certain amount of vitamins, minerals, and other nutrients. Excessive amounts are eliminated in the urine and feces. Taking nutrients in excess of body needs is not "insurance," but IS enervating and burdensome to the system. When nutritional organization and balance is not achieved, the body exhibits symptoms in its attempt to regain homeostasis.

Building health is a harmonious body effort and not a defensive action. Drugs and supplements are tolerated more over time but provide nothing but a false facade of excitation, not health.

Taking supplements cripples the system's powers of synthesis and, after a time, as with drugs, the person finds they must have recourse to an increased supplement intake to obtain the same illusionary feeling of well-being. In the meantime so long as lifestyle is not aligned with our biological mandate, no healing has taken place and internal deterioration proceeds unabated.

Where there is NO demand for the production of a body secretion or product, the body ceases its generation. When supplements are substituted for nutrients that are normally liberated from foods as a result of a biological process, the time soon arrives when supplement-dependency may occur—the metabolism atrophies and no longer manufactures or efficiently metabolizes nutrients that are vital to life.

Without artificial supplementation, health rapidly deteriorates. Meanwhile, no "cure" has been affected, and the lack, instead, continues to reassert itself. In this case, a fast usually renormalizes metabolism and restores the body's ability to obtain required nutrients from foods for which we are biologically suited.

Organic vs. Inorganic Nutrients—the Body Knows the Difference

One group of vital nutrients required throughout the body are the mineral salts. Minerals are a part of every cell, tissue, organ, and system—being especially concentrated in the bones, teeth, hair, and nails. Without minerals, blood alkalinity and other body fluids would be in extreme jeopardy because proper mineral presence is required to sustain proper pH, as well as proper viscosity (fluidity) and salinity (saltiness) of all systemic fluids.

Our body depends upon only *naturally* chelated minerals, those organically organized within living food molecules. Inorganic molecules are lifeless, whereas plant food molecules use sunlight to transform inorganic salts into complex protein/amino acid bound molecules which our system can efficiently utilize in its metabolic processes.

Humans cannot eat directly of the soil and live. We cannot take into our physiology inorganic elements and build a healthy body for these poison our system. But when taken up as food by the plant and combined into complex organic formulations and reorganized into widely diverse forms of vegetable matter, these become digestible and provide us with rich nutriment for sustaining life.

Synthetically derived supplements advertised as "organic" are neither digestible nor metabolizable except, perhaps, those derived through bacterial action. The body is stimulated by synthetic or so-called "organic" supplements just as if caffeine, alcohol or other drugs had been taken since most supplements are derived from rocks, soils, sea water, or ores that are unusable and poisonous.

Selenium, iodine, and chromium for instance are trace

minerals, essential to the body. But in inorganic form these are very toxic and even bear the "skull and crossbones" insignia on their commercial preparations. As elaborated by plant life via photosynthesis, however, we can readily use their ORGANIC forms but the human body rejects *inorganic salts* because it has no mechanism to use them.

It is futile to dose the body with isolated nutrient supplements, whether artificially chelated or not, *since* ***the body requires all nutrients in proper synergistic proportion to one another.***

When consumed "out of balance," so to speak, inorganic minerals are rejected by the human body. If they cannot be promptly removed, they remain in body fluids or are deposited as a precipitate in the form of stones or plaque wherever convenient, although remaining an impediment to efficient physiological function.

Common table salt, minerals used to "enrich" and "fortify" overly processed manufactured foods, nutritional supplements, denatured nutrients from cooked foods, antacid preparations, tap water, mineralized water, supplements, etc., are harmful in this regard. Other than fresh air, pure water, and sunshine, the body cannot utilize anything whatsoever except **ORGANIC** compounds as found in our natural foods.

INORGANIC substances, on the other hand, clog up our circulation if not eliminated. They combine with body fluids, oils, and waste materials to form plaque or stones which saturate our vascular system, or are abnormally deposited within our joints, muscles, lymphatic system, and various organs, especially the gallbladder and kidneys.

The body also treats herbal supplements just as it does other stimulants—by rushing them to the nearest exit with all the haste, vigor, and energy it can muster. In taking herbal concoctions, we only add to the body's burdens. Instead of directing its energies exclusively to detoxification, it must also eliminate the herbal poison as well and, in the process, the body is hampered in its self-healing efforts.

Natural Hygiene vs. Modern Medicine

Hygienic Self-Health Care recognizes that we do not require special remedies when illness strikes since wholesome materials and influences continue to be wholesome when sick, just as they are during health. The supply of wholesome factors in disease must be in keeping with the body's capacity to utilize them.

A true science of Health Care rests solely upon correct principles of physiology. What does this imply in practice in both the art of healing and the art of living? Simply, aligning ourselves with our natural mandate—for we cannot depart from our needs without incurring disease.

To regain health, the sick need to regain alignment with their biological requisites—just as to preserve health, those who are well, need to maintain such alignment.

And yet, we see just the opposite. The world behaves in accordance with a medical rationale that *wholesome* agents are only adapted to those who are well, while ***un****wholesome* agents are NECESSARY for those who are diseased.

The medical system endeavors to make the sick well by administering poisonous drugs which make even healthy persons sick, whereas Natural Hygiene restores the sick to health by the means that preserve health within those who are well in the first place. Why experiment with a host of "remedies" when the study of physiological cause and effect is called for?

The public must be taught to prevent disease by avoiding its causes rather than attempting to cure illness by administering the causes of other illnesses. If people were educated thoroughly with the principles of physiology and Hygiene, there would be little need for physicians since their job would be fulfilled—health of the masses.

The means to restore health are the same factors of food, air, water, sunshine, activity, rest, sleep, cleanliness, and emotional poise upon which life depend and NOT in the anti-vital drugging measures of the physician. Rather, in the normal wholesome conditions and materials of Hygiene are located the influences and essentials out of which health is generated.

And this means health of the whole being not merely some part of it. Hygiene, therefore, is no tool of the medical specialist who would rather treat the heart or liver while largely ignoring the rest of the system.

The effects of Hygienic Self-Health Care are entirely in the direction of natural growth and, consequently, are of a permanent nature so long as the essentials of health are continuously provided. As such, their effects are quite distinct from those that are only *apparently* beneficial which result from medical treatment of symptoms only and not of their underlying cause.

When injury or disease occurs, modern medicine generally takes an overly invasive, aggressive approach that often poses more risk than the problem at hand. Drugs and surgery are often directed at symptoms of disease, rather than the ACTUAL problem itself.

It must be determined what factors are responsible for the symptoms, and then remove the causes in order to best support the body's self-healing mechanisms. If all health professionals would practice in like manner, the medical profession and related pharmaceutical industries as we know them would be out of business.

In summary:

- *Hygienic practitioners* attend to the organic requirements of the body to **rebuild health**, whereas *physicians* attempt to **"cure" disease**;
- *Hygienic practitioners* remove harmful substances and influences through **education** in what comprises a biologically adapted lifestyle regime, whereas *physicians* **ignore harmful lifestyle routines** and attempt to immunize against their consequences, or to palliate their symptoms; and, finally,
- *Hygienic practitioners* **teach** the essentials of health to establish **self-sufficiency** in matters of health care, whereas *physicians* indirectly assume responsibility to "make the patient better," creating **dependency** in matters of health care.

The True Nature of Disease and the *Modus Operandi* of Medicinal Substances

As discussed earlier, the phenomenon of "curing" and so-called "side-effects" that result when medicinal remedies, herbs, and supplements are taken, are actually evidence of vital resistance of the body against the drug, whereby the system expedites the drug's expulsion. In no way are these "remedial actions" as commonly supposed.

Rather, it is the modus operandi of the living organism in action. The modus operandi of drugs is a misnomer, since the notion that drugs "act" is not in accord with how physiology operates. The rationale of the effects of all "medicines" is inseparably connected with life and in no way distinct from it.

For some 3,000 years, philosophers, scientists, and medical men have sought an understanding of the *modus operandi* of medicinal drugs; the nature of disease; and the precise relationship between drugs, disease, and the healing power of nature.

Disease today is still listed as one of the "seven modern mysteries." While most pharmacology texts contain brief efforts explaining drug action, none are satisfactory under the scrutiny of the laws of physiology. To the medical field, drug action is as much a mystery as the nature of disease itself (even the "action" of aspirin, for example, remains a mystery). As they were in the days of Hippocrates, drugs are still thought of as antagonistic forces to those responsible for disease.

Even though the essential nature of disease is unknown, medical authorities incessantly drug disease as though they know all about it. *But how can a successful means of dealing with illness and treating the sick be devised when it is not understood?* Knowledge of the essential nature of disease must provide the very foundation of any scientific care of the sick.

The Hygienic Health-Care System *does profess* to understand the nature of disease and the apparent "actions" of drugs—and from this understanding, all drugs are rejected.

The principles and practices of Hygienic Health-Care have never been written in medical books, nor taught in medical schools, nor recognized by the medical profession. Instead of research to validate the science of Hygiene, medicine seems busily engaged in trying to dispose of it. Rather than condemning and questioning it, would it not be worthwhile to seek the true causes of increasing disease throughout our populace?

Even though contradictory to "modern" medicine, the fundamental principles on which Hygiene is based are demonstrably in harmony with the laws of physiology.

Consequences of Violating Our Natural Mandate

Actually, it is impossible to "break or violate" a law of physiology but we *can* choose to ignore the essentials of health and suffer the consequences or to observe and follow our natural mandate and reap the benefits.

Nature has not provided remedies for disease. Nature has, however, provided consequences for partaking in actions that occasion illness. To create and maintain health, we need to observe the requirements of life and live within their limitations or suffer the results.

For example, *if we overeat or eat biologically improper foods, if we ingest poisons* or in any way fail to supply the body with its needs or subject it to inappropriate conditions, then the degree of disharmony experienced is determined by the level of impairment to our health. *The sun*, which nourishes our body, will enervate and damage it if overexposed. *Exercise* is essential for utilization and appropriation of nutrients by the body, but overexertion causes exhaustion, impairing our ability to assimilate foodstuffs. In this way, the essentials of life are understood to have limitations which we must abide by.

Living in accord with our needs means conducting our daily affairs such that we live consciously—aware of how our choices contribute to our continuing health or toward disease. The function of Natural Hygiene is to provide knowledge of the essentials of health, rather than trying to find means of circumventing natural laws of well-being.

Most people are brainwashed to believe they can continue abusing the body, and that drugs and chemicals will cure them. *This, in turn, takes away from the body's ability to heal itself.* THE SECRET IS TO TEACH PEOPLE HOW TO TAKE CHARGE OF THEIR HEALTH THROUGH PROPER NUTR-

ITION, PROPER EXERCISE, AND THROUGH CULTIVATING MENTAL AND EMOTIONAL WELL-BEING.

This manner of living responsibly is challenging and requires diligence—especially within the context of our pathological society. Do the best job possible, as animals in nature do instinctively without any special knowledge or training. In this way, we align ourselves with the essentials of life and reap the rewards—healthful living, along with the realization that WE are largely in control of our own health destiny.

Chapter 13

AWAKENING OUR SELF HEALING BODY: PROVIDING THE OPTIMAL CONDITIONS FOR "SPONTANEOUS RECOVERY"

Healing is *entirely* a biological process just as is respiration, nutrition, excretion, and other body activities. The body is a completely self-healing organism, and this healing takes place to the degree that our physiological needs are provided for.

This organic recuperation and reconstruction requires no goads to action to continue the vital changes towards a salubrious state. Our task is to establish the best possible conditions so that the body may conduct the healing process quickly and efficiently without obstacles hindering its progress.

The body is fully capable of correcting all internal imbalances and will automatically do so as soon as disease causes are removed (and sometimes before causes are removed if a life threatening state exists).

The body actively pursues total health at all times resonant with its present capabilities. If allowed to do so, the body will detoxify itself without the use of any external agents. The body is a perfect, self-sufficient healing system which can, under normal circumstances, instigate the return to health (barring any genetic disorder exists).

The body ALWAYS aims for improvement by trying to produce health unless our interference is too great. Only then do we fail to recover and further degenerate towards chronic disease—unless we change to an improved lifestyle and do something constructive to reverse the downhill process. Due to poor living and eating habits, toxins introduced into the body cause disease. When the diet is sufficiently wholesome or when food is withheld, the body can eliminate these toxins and restore health.

Illness is the result of unhealthful living. Health is restored by removing these causes, and by supplying the conditions for health. Drugless health practitioners do not dispense drugs or contaminants to an already toxic organism but rely on natural means which utilize the body's self-sufficient ability to heal.

Healing is a normal biological process which continually functions both during sickness and health and that results from the orderly operations and regular forces of life working with agents and substances that bear a normal relation to the living organism.

The body’s success at self-healing depends completely upon the removal of the cause of its ills. No healing can take place without removal of cause, followed by supplying the body with its basic needs so it may correct the condition.

Health is the organism's natural tendency—**we do not have to MAKE the body healthy, we only have to LIVE healthfully.** In doing so, ask yourself the following questions:

1. Am I eating a biologically proper diet—mostly fruits, vegetables, nuts and seeds in their raw, natural fresh state?
2. Am I eating only when hungry, and then not over-eating?
3. Do I consume the purest water (distilled) available?
4. Is the air I breathe fresh and clean?
5. Do I get sufficient rest and sleep?
6. Do I get enough exercise?
7. Am I exposed to sunlight at least a few minutes daily?
8. Am I constructively handling stressful situations?

To return health to the body, it must be provided with its requirements. But first those substances, influences, practices, and poor lifestyle habits which beget disease must be discontinued.

To Re-Establish Self-Healing, Remove the Causes of Disease

All illness must be caused. Almost always, cause is initiated by the person suffering or it can be avoided. Unless cause is eliminated, the body continues to degenerate. **In re-creating health, then, two things must be done: remove**

the causes of disease; and establish the conditions of health.

When cause is removed, body wisdom takes over and moves the system towards health as soon as our basic organic needs are met. When all of the conditions of health are supplied, the body never fails to work for the general good of the entire organism.

There is nothing outside of the body that has any power whatsoever to heal—there is no outside intelligence or guidelines which can fully assess and determine the complete extent of the body's needs. There are no technologies or machines that can accurately determine the causes of a particular ailment.

Nothing outside the body can fabricate blood, lymph, and other body fluids, and direct them to where they are most needed. There is no outside substance which can correctly evaluate our physiological circumstances and decide which cells are to be replaced or retained, or where new cells may be needed most to enhance systemic function and meet structural needs. **Only the body possesses the residual potential, power and intelligence to heal itself, and will do so when favorable conditions are provided.**

Healing also depends upon the amount of vitality possessed to power the transition to a healthful state. Through proper care, the human body is automatically subject to positive, constructive change.

Healing takes time, however, just as the evolution of disease takes time to lay the body low. We must have patience and let the system accomplish its necessary work. The body will do its own metabolic balancing and will eventually discard the putrid decaying accumulations it has been unable to previously eliminate.

The organism never remains in a static position—it will move either forward or backward depending on whether we answer systemic requirements. As our energy level rises or falls, the movement "uphill or downhill" accelerates. So once we consciously embark on the transition to biologically proper living, we must persevere and soon the result will be an efficiently functioning, peaceful body.

So long as life remains, the ability of the human body to heal and improve itself ALWAYS exists to some extent. Cellular replication, secretion of body fluids, and excretion of metabolic wastes continues non-stop so long as the force of life exists—although it becomes more feeble as functioning power wanes due to subsequent wasting of our powers and energies.

Health is natural and normal, illness is not. The body always strives to maintain homeostasis. If illness manifests, it means the body has not been provided the best circumstances for maintaining a balanced state of health and instead has been overwhelmed with toxins. A "healing crisis" is initiated to rid itself of the toxic burden.

At this point, if causes of disease are removed and requirements for health provided, illness will no longer progress and health will be regained. On the other hand, if symptoms are palliated by drugging, the toxic overload will not be discharged. More serious illness will ensue later in life.

When Sick, "Leave the Body *Intelligently* Alone"

There are no "magic bullets"—our body's inner "know-how" is in charge, not our intellect, whims, or wishes. Any effort to control body function amounts to abnormal interference which is potentially injurious to the organism.

Our drugging practices are based on conjectures about what we erroneously believe the body should be doing, or what we think it needs when ill . **In times of illness, LEAVE THE BODY INTELLIGENTLY ALONE and establish the external conditions of health based on the body's**

capabilities and let the body self-purify.

All treatments and so-called "healing substances" impede health restoration by adding more burden with which the body has to contend. But as long as we cooperate with the body's inner "know-how" by supplying the best conditions for healing, improved health will occur. Unhealthful lifestyle practices ALWAYS demand a toll on the body, but improvement in health will always follow in the wake of correct modes of living.

Diseases will not occur unless we cause them. The only way not to cause disease is to live in accordance with the principles that govern the health of our body.

Given the conditions of health, the body will rebuild well-being in nearly all cases. Establish the conditions more favorable to health and leave the body intelligently alone. When sick, if the body cannot restore itself under the most favorable conditions for recovery, then it is irremediable. Adopt the attitude that the body is its own panacea in ALL cases.

One of the prime dictates of the Hygienic philosophy is non-interference with the body. Treating various disease symptoms differently because they appear in different areas of the body is senseless. Almost all diseases should be treated the same way—by non-interference. A thorough-going rest under tranquil surroundings constitutes the best healing environment.

The more unhampered the body is in its restorative efforts, the more that the natural "cure" is most effective due to the body's intrinsic power to heal itself. In health, the body needs proper food, vigorous activity, and adequate rest, sleep, and sunshine. In disease, the body needs extra rest and sleep in order to regain normal functioning. To meet this need we temporarily cease eating and exercising and conserve digestive and muscular energies.

We can furnish the body with the highest-quality food when needed, or withhold food altogether when it is not desired. We can exercise or rest the body, give it fresh air and sunshine but other than this, all we can do is intelligently wait and not become alarmed by healing symptoms nor suppress them with drugs or medicinal herbs.

The body is self-healing and its regenerative powers must be given full reign without interference. Anything done to "cure" or stop the body's regenerative actions are impediments that only thwart the system's cleansing efforts. Leave the body alone and it will regain normal function.

Because of misunderstandings about the nature of the human body and its normal functioning, people routinely suffer ill health. This suffering, however, is unnecessary.

Disease action on the part of the body occasions suffering because of adverse conditions that have been imposed upon the system. The suffering occurs NOT because of incorrect action by the body but because the body is struggling to free itself from impending dangers resulting from poor lifestyle habits of misuse and abuse.

Disease evolves initially from our constant reaction to stress in our environment and from physiological/metabolic responses to our daily enervating and life depleting habits. These influences strain either the physical body, the mind, or the emotions and we become enervated.

Slowly, cellular toxic overload increases, leading to cellular constipation and inefficient systemic elimination. Metabolic waste is retained over a long period as the kidneys, bowels, lungs, and other eliminative organs lose their efficiency from being constantly overworked. Toxemia is generated and the disease response follows—first acute crises and then chronic, degenerative conditions unless lifestyle changes are implemented.

The Vital Body Continually Strives For Health

Ideally, we should live so as to not foul up the body in the first place. If, through stress and other uncontrollable circumstances, the body dams-up its metabolic wastes, do not pollute it further by ingesting foreign or unmetabolizable substances.

Instead, the individual must be left alone and provided with the requisites of health so that body intelligence may best marshall its resources. In this way, the pendulum of energy can swing once more in the opposite direction, towards recuperation and re-invigoration.

In our modern environment, the human body is exposed to many toxins daily. Under normal circumstances, the body is able to eliminate them rapidly via our eliminative organs: the kidneys, liver, lungs, and the skin. But when the level of toxins rises to where the body is overloaded, our vital energy drops and the organs of elimination are unable to maintain functional efficiency. The body's internal environment becomes unstable.

At this point remedial steps must be taken to reduce toxemia. Either we recognize the mild functional disturbance and decide to fast and rest to speedily restore functional efficiency to the body, or the organism itself will take remedial steps and institute disease. At this point, we should cooperate with the body's cleansing efforts by undergoing a thorough, complete rest until the system regains the ability to eliminate body wastes through normal channels.

Profound Rest Is Best

The ONLY source of healing is your own body, and the only way we can help this process is by providing ideal conditions for the implementation

of its own self-healing power.

The human body BEST heals itself, purifies itself, and repairs damages from injuries caused by toxins under the condition where complete rest is obtained. Deep rest is needed during healing because the body must recuperate its depleted nerve energy and thereby increase its residual vitality in order to further conduct and complete the healing crisis at hand.

When the body exhibits acute symptoms, do not take drugs or herbal remedies. If cold symptoms, skin eruptions, rashes, headache, stomach ache, hay fever, flu or pain symptoms of any kind manifest the best thing to do is REST.

The ENTIRE BODY needs profound physiological rest —the muscles, organs, glands, digestive system, and our mental faculties. The system is in a state of extreme enervation and, in order to heal, all available bodily energies must be directed solely to the task. No food, only pure water and bed rest is the proper dietary routine. The body is then provided with ideal conditions to redirect its energies to the reparative process and the system begins to cleanse and revitalize its physiological capacities.

In this way, the body removes the morbid internal waste material; dissolves excess fat which clogs the system; autolyzes cysts, tumors, and abnormal growths; and, in short, rebuilds a healthy and a superbly functioning organism by using all the fundamental requisites of organic existence. Once this is accomplished, symptoms depart since our blood and fluids are no longer polluted. They are free-flowing, pure, and service the needs of each cell and tissue.

In disease, our aim is to cooperate with the body in its efforts to restore normal functioning so that the life-sustaining processes of nutrition and drainage can effectively be carried out. The body behaves in essentially the same way in a state of health as it does in a state of ill-health—only the conditions change, and the body then redistributes its energy and resources as necessary to recover a state of normality.

Once you realize that the system as a whole is toxic, there is only one way to constructively serve the organism—by fasting, resting, and, thereafter, *healthful living.* Once this condition is restored, high-level health and freedom from disease is the natural result.

The Controlled Fast

Fasting is perhaps the safest, most effective means of correcting the maladies of the body—NOT as a curative measure, but more as an incidental result of an improvement in one's lifestyle.

Healing is a normal body process which continues constantly throughout life in relation to the amount of energy available. By fasting, we fully cooperate with the body's self-healing powers which enable the necessary elimination of toxins to proceed with minimum discomfort and maximum speed, as the body saves all the energy usually consumed during eating, digesting, assimilating, and absorbing food particles and uses it, instead, to cleanse and repair itself.

Throughout the animal kingdom, abstinence from eating when sick is actually instinctual. Even domesticated animals will sit by their water dishes and partake of little, or nothing else, until the self-limited illness subsides. When WE fall ill, our appetite similarly subsides or disappears altogether and distilled water is all that should be ingested until symptoms of the disease/healing process end.

During the fast, as we abstain from all physical, emotional, sensory, and digestive activities, all available body energy including that of the nervous system as well as biochemical and mechanical energies can be redirected to internal purification. A controlled withdrawal of food for a reasonable period of time allows the body to revitalize and carry out its healing processes.

During the period of abstinence, the body needs to devote NO energy whatsoever to digestion and absorption of food—this energy is devoted instead to elimination of waste, tissue constipation, and toxemia all of which interfere with the body's normal metabolic functioning. Under no other condition can the body so quickly and efficiently detoxify and restore itself.

During the fast, the chemistry of the body's fluids and secretions undergo rapid change and return to a normal, healthy state.

If at any time during this cleansing drugs are taken to suppress detoxification symptoms, the toxic matter will be re-directed back into the system, increasing toxicosis and making the healing crisis more severe. The body must then initiate a more desperate attempt to eliminate its overload through more distressful means.

The body's ability to heal can be enhanced if the "remedies" and causes that have built disease are removed. The body must be given an opportunity to eliminate its toxic accumulation via the fast and then maintain a purer blood chemistry through a change in diet and lifestyle. In this manner, the system becomes younger in physiological condition—its functions are qualitatively improved, its structures repaired, and its fitness to live increased.

In fact, as long as we are alive, the body *constantly* undergoes a process of regeneration. Cells and tissues are renewed daily, delaying old age and early death as much as possible despite the abuses we constantly impose on the system. Fasting enables the processes of renewal to out-distance the processes of degeneration. The result is a higher standard of health.

While fasting, the healing process is not *qualitatively* different than in normal times, although the *quantity* of actions differ as healing IS greatly accelerated. In most cases this involves the body removing accumulated waste materials that interfere with normal cellular functioning.

The fast itself does nothing but provide ideal conditions during which the body can effectively rebuild its health by rapidly normalizing itself during which time, healing is concentrated and consolidated. ***Fasting is a tool—it is not a "cure."*** As such, fasting should not be used as a crutch to fall back on whenever we choose to live unhealthfully, for this will further enervate the system.

Fasting is but one part of an entire healthy lifestyle that will maintain health when incorporated properly into our routine (perhaps one long weekend from Friday afternoon to Sunday evening every six to eight weeks).

Between fasts, the body's needs should be provided for, including proper food and water, adequate sunshine and fresh air, rest and sleep, and emotional poise. Fasting for health restoration is the one extraordinary measure EVERYONE should incorporate into their lifestyle within the context of our pathogenic society.

While fasting, the body effects a remission of toxicosis with the least amount of damage to the living organism. At all times, the body protects its systemic integrity. This is why the body does not suddenly discharge all the toxic and morbid accumulations "in one complete sweep," so to speak. Instead, they are removed in proportion to the rate and manner in which they were accumulated.

Keep in mind, that the body does NOT have unlimited powers of healing. The body's ability to successfully heal during a fast is determined by how much tissue destruction has occurred over the duration of toxemia, and how vigorous the body's healing powers are.

As we age, the powers of healing diminish. Adults, for instance, rarely display the physiological vigor seen in the infant whose body is relatively pure, toleration low, and resistance high.

When provided the conditions necessary to generate health the body spontaneously begins restoring itself to normality to the extent of its residual potential.

Problems that are irremediable, however, like amputated parts, excised organs, and degenerative conditions will not mend but can be improved. In some cases where the body has suffered irreparable organic damage, the system will not have sufficient vitality to completely heal, although improvement in disease conditions will virtually always be experienced.

When the chronically diseased individual fasts, a marked acceleration of detoxification occurs. Long standing symptoms often disappear. After a biologically correct mode of living is established, the body will evolve into a more enhanced state of health relative to the residual vitality maintainable by the impaired organism. AT LEAST partial recovery from asthma, diabetes, high blood pressure, heart disorders, various tumors, and numerous other diseases is thereby achieved.

While some consider the fast a panacea, it will NOT enable the body to restore many forms of organic degeneration, although improvement in health and general condition will always occur.

When the resources and powers of the body fail to restore health under the most favorable conditions, the degenerated state is irremediable. EVERYONE can benefit by the employment of healthful practices, however, within the context of their condition.

The time to fast, therefore, is BEFORE the body becomes debilitated by chronic disease. If we fast when symptoms of acute disease first express themselves and then adhere to a more healthy lifestyle, chronic degenerative disease will not develop.

Often, the body's healing efforts as exhibited through acute disease symptoms are suppressed and palliated by various drugs. In this case, the body is never allowed to eliminate its toxic overload from years of incorrect eating and unhealthful lifestyle practices. Due to this constant suppression and continued violation of our biological needs, degenerative disease eventually takes hold.

If seriously ill, a therapeutic fast of between 14-30 days on distilled water alone may be necessary since pathological conditions may not respond to dietary and lifestyle changes in any reasonable time frame (if at all) without abstinence and the focused healing which accompanies it.

An impaired organism needs to recuperate and then be fed only those foods which provide maximum nutritional value in return for the work the body must perform in processing the foodstuffs.

The body is incredibly provident and intelligent in its self-preserving capabilities. Under normal conditions (in the absence of metabolic imbalances, nutritional deficiencies, or atrophy of a vital organ, gland, or tissue), the body has plenty of reserves automatically set aside for crisis situations.

This is why the body can abstain from food for extended periods, allowing our reserve fund to supply our nutrient needs while energy is redirected toward ejecting poisons. As the fast progresses, the body explores and then utilizes its reserves of life-sustaining nutrients that are salvaged and absorbed by our cells.

Under the condition of the fast, the body initially uses its most efficient fuel of all—its own fat reserves—AFTER first exhausting the contents of the intestinal tract.

After two to three days, the body slowly begins autolyzing growths (tumors, warts, cysts, etc.) and eventually divests itself of most, if not all, alien substances including plaque in arteries and veins; stones in the gallbladder and kidneys; ossification materials in the brain, feet, joints, and lower back; and less vital cells, errant cells, and even cancer cells to some degree.

While fasting the body breaks down and burns for energy these non-essential substances. After two to six weeks in the non-obese individual, this process is completed. When the fat reserves have been eliminated, the fast is complete. Starvation begins unless food is eaten at this point, as the body then begins to break down essential tissues for energy production.

"Elimination Diets"

Due to increases in free-floating toxins throughout the general circulation (including the lymph and bloodstream) that had previously been stored away inside fatty tissues, certain impaired individuals should not fast before undergoing initial detoxification via an "elimination diet" of mostly fresh juicy fruit.

Diets that are not stressful to the body allow it to more efficiently perform its eliminative functions. Such "elimination diets" of fruit are sometimes useful when intense symptoms require cessation of normal food intake but it is not possible to fast and take prolonged bed rest.

Once on an elimination diet that is very easily digested the body's digestive task is immensely simplified, it can devote its energies to restoration and cleansing. Even though long-term benefits of the fast will not be accomplished, a temporary juice and/or fruit diet may be indicated at times depending on individual circumstances.

Elimination diets are low in protein, carbohydrates and, fats which cause cells to use stored reserves to meet their metabolic requirements. During the elimination diet, the body can eliminate toxic material and accumulated wastes but not nearly as efficiently or thoroughly as during a fast. The body derives greater benefit from one week of a complete fast than from two or three weeks of an elimination diet.

Symptoms of Detoxification and Healing

As the body detoxifies during fasting or while undergoing an eliminative diet, symptoms may arise at the onset as our body chemistry re-adjusts itself. As curative, health-building changes begin and the body normalizes, changes are initiated which may prove disconcerting at times due to the system's accelerated purification efforts.

At first, you may feel quite hungry, faint, and weak. Weight loss and minor discomforts such as headaches and unpleasant stomach sensations may occur as the system repairs systemic damage and re-orients itself away from denatured, devitalized foods.

Weight loss occurs since the body temporarily discards waste more rapidly than new tissue is formed. Old obstructive material that has been stored in the tissues and joints is flushed out—all signs of the body building health. Symptoms such as headache, nausea, weight loss, etc., should not be suppressed or viewed negatively since this evidence of cleansing are the signs of a vital body working diligently to re-establish well-being.

In the process of health regeneration when a better diet is implemented, the body's first phase of action is recuperation. **During this initial phase (lasting from ten days to several weeks), *the health seeker may feel weaker and sicker than on the old, poorer quality diet.*** This is because the body's vital energies usually within the peripheral muscles and extremities begin to move toward the internal organs and tissues to start intensive reconstruction.

Energy is utilized to flush out toxins and to remove cellular contamination. (Actually during this time, there is INCREASED energy but at this phase of detoxification, the mind does not interpret it as such). Headaches and nausea may be noted due to withdrawal from stimulating, inferior food but these temporary phenomena will soon be replaced by greater stamina and enhanced well-being.

This shunting of power to our internal organs produces a feeling of less energy in the muscles. Once again, the body's functioning power is actually increasing but most of it is being used for rebuilding the vital organs and less is immediately available for the musculature. **This weakness is not true weakness, but merely an internal re-deploying of bodily resources.** The need for rest and sleep increases during this crucial phase of health regeneration.

If stimulants are used at this point, the body will abort its regenerative efforts and we defeat its very purpose. Have faith (based on understanding) and wait it out—increased strength and vigor will return and will exceed what was experienced previously. Success hinges on relaxing and taking it easy at this point. Coast in your work obligations until your "out of the woods" so to speak.

Every drug used, whether prescribed, over-the-counter, or "recreational" leaves its mark upon the body. As the body regains health through a progressively more biologically correct lifestyle, drug deposits that were stored away within fatty tissues and organs are released into the bloodstream for removal.

Since a combination of past drug deposits may enter the circulation at once, disconcerting symptoms may express themselves in a series of rashes as they leave through the skin. The release of toxins may occasion certain symptoms such as headaches or nausea, but they do not indicate that the cleansing crisis is harmful, nor do symptoms foretell a worsening condition. Instead, they indicate that the body is undergoing a much needed internal cleansing.

Symptoms are temporary and, although uncomfortable,

they will vanish as toxins are removed from the body. Drug detoxification may be a lengthy process but it will be aided by fasting and a diet high in fresh juicy fruits.

As we continue on the improved lifestyle and higher quality diet, the body continues this process known as "retracing." The finer nutritive materials consumed are used to clear the body of poorer quality materials, and to improve the body's structure and functional capacity.

For instance, excess bile is purged from the liver and gallbladder and is sent to the intestines for elimination. Plaque and cholesterol are moved out of the arteries, veins, and capillaries. Accumulated fecal deposits and bowel masses are removed; arthritic deposits in the joints and calcium deposits in the kidneys and gallbladder are broken down and eliminated. Fat deposits are slowly dissolved. All this continues until the body is rebuilt and purified.

During "retracing," the body throws out poisons held internally more rapidly than ever now that the body has more power to do so—which in large part, comes from discontinuing those hard-to-digest meals.

The body, however, will not kill itself or allow healing to progress as to cause life-threatening discomfort. The body is wise enough to accelerate the healing crisis as rapidly as possible. This may involve MAJOR purging and ejection of literally pounds of accumulated toxins from decades of improper eating and living practices that are dumped into the circulation to be eliminated.

The toxins being discarded save the body from more serious, future disease including hepatitis, arthritis, kidney disorders, blood diseases, cardiovascular problems, and even cancer, any of which could result if the poisons are retained.

The Body Does Not "Turn On Itself" In Times of Disease

Occasionally, "scientific" articles are published describing how the body"s "immune system turns on itself" and attacks its own domain—ulcers and arthritis being examples. This is nonsense, however.

What the body does in arthritis is store toxic debris (including calcium-urate crystals) within the joints as a life-preserving measure until they can be safely removed.

In the case of ulcers, millions of cells are destroyed in creating and autolyzing an exit to the skins surface as in boils, acne, etc., in order to remove deadly accumulations that pose greater problems to the general economy. In each case, the body acts for the greater good of its some 100 trillion cells even though tissue is temporarily sacrificed in the process.

Because we do not understand the body is no reason to blame it for the problems we suffer. Rather than a breakdown in our defense mechanisms in these cases, we are instead witnessing the body choosing a lesser evil in order to preserve its functional integrity at the highest possible level under adverse circumstances. Just because a local defense mechanism has been temporarily overruled by our overall body intelligence, does NOT mean that our genetic endowment has "turned against us."

When our intellect and power of choice defies our instincts in pursuing a lifestyle contrary to our biological mandate, the cause of disease lies with the pathogenic practices of the sufferer. The body commands the sacrifice of a localized area to aid in remedying the danger, which can be speedily enhanced by fasting, biologically correct diet, adequate exercise, and other beneficent lifestyle factors. Mixed up genes is not the problem—mixed up priorities and lifestyle patterns are.

Lifestyle Improvements and Initial Weightloss—Catabolism is Followed By Anabolism

When diet and lifestyle improvements are made and when higher quality food is consumed, when we get more rest, more exercise, and more fresh air and sunshine, remarkable things begin to happen in the body.

When nutrients consumed are of higher quality than the tissues which compose the body, the physiology begins to make room for the superior materials which it uses to create new, healthier tissue.

Spontaneously, the organism begins to discard and recycle all lower-grade cells and tissues—all usable recycled materials are incorporated along with the incoming top-grade nutrients and these are collectively used to literally construct a new, healthier body.

As healthy living continues, the body's biological evolutionary process renews and revitalizes each successive generation of cells, such that they are healthier than the preceding generation.

When we improve the conditions and environment of the body, it starts improving itself. Initially, it goes into a *catabolic* stage where it breaks down inferior tissues and ejects toxic materials. Depending on the individual and on the approach, whether fasting or on an elimination diet, this may last for weeks or months before the body pretty much completes the cleansing and starts the *anabolic* process of rebuilding new, healthy, vibrantly robust tissue.

During this initial catabolic breakdown phase of metabolism, the accent is on elimination, or the breakdown of tissues as garbage deposits throughout the body are removed. At this point, accumulated waste materials are discarded more rapidly than new tissue is built from the higher quality food ingested. Weightloss is experienced which persists until the second phase of metabolism—STABILIZATION—is reached.

During the stabilization phase of metabolism, body weight remains more or less stable as the amount of waste material being discarded each day equals the quantity of tissue being formed and replaced via the more vital food supply. This takes place after excess obstructions have been removed from the tissues. Stabilization persists for a while and is followed by the third phase of metabolism called ANABOLISM.

Anabolism is the body's building stage wherein weight increases even though the diet contains fewer calories than before. At this point, most interfering wastes have been discarded.

The newly formed body tissues are more durable, higher quality, and do not as readily break down as the lower quality tissue did. Also, new tissues are formed faster than before due to increased assimilation and increased digestive enzyme efficiency made possible by the cessation of improper food intake.

When the fluids of the body are kept reasonably pure and clean by adhering to the Hygienic lifestyle, we can maintain a high level of health and have amazing vitality as compared with the rest of our diseased populace—EVEN IN TODAY'S STRESSED AND POLLUTED ENVIRONMENT.

This healthy state is best preserved with an occasional cleansing fast of comparatively short duration . After the fast, eat predominantly of those foods to which we are physiologically suited: raw fruits, vegetables, nuts and seeds in compatible combinations in conjunction with a moderate exercise program.

The Proper "Prescription" is Healthful Living

There is only one way back to good health—HEALTHFUL LIVING, meaning the observance of our physiological needs. Health is the condition wherein we have complete function of all our faculties. This state of wholeness and harmonious operation of all body organs and mental faculties represents a condition of optimal development.

Health proceeds ONLY from the orderly biological processes of the body. The human body always tends to grow toward improved health when provided with the proper tools and influences. By employing healthful measures you do your body a true service instead of further destroying health with pills and medical modalities.

A healthy body seeks to preserve itself. *The sensation of wellness IS sensational and health maintenance gains our conscious support as a consequence as we directly experience the fruits of our lifestyle choices.* A sick body, on the other hand, is an intoxicated body which often hurtles toward self-destruction through unhealthful lifestyle behaviors, negative thought patterns, and incoherent action.

It is much easier to KEEP the body in health than it is to restore health once it has become impaired. Likewise, it is much easier to maintain healthful lifestyle habits than it is to break destructive patterns after they have become fixed.

The choice is ours. Health is ONLY produced by *consciously* living healthfully. This is why, once health is restored, the body's well-being should be preserved through the study and practice of Hygienic Health Care.

Once you understand and trust in your body's ability to heal itself, the unpleasant symptoms in those who are seriously ill also become understood and bearable, and not a source of fear and misgiving. Let the body perform its health restoration work at its own pace. The body *alone* is capable of performing all of its required healing functions.

Health is Built Gradually, Not Overnight

Once diet and lifestyle are improved, DO NOT think or expect to feel better each day until death. Body detoxification is a lifelong process—even in a state of pristine health. Our body always strives for a higher state of health and is constantly eliminating toxins as soon as our metabolism forms them.

Consequently, some cleansing symptoms may occur from time to time even after a high state of well-being has been established. Symptoms, however, will be of much shorter duration and much lower intensity since the body is already relatively pure. Instead of a cold lasting for a week, it may only last for one to two days, or you may only notice a temporary cleansing lasting for a few hours overnight instead of over extended periods as is usually the norm.

The body's purification efforts are cyclical in nature, and health returns in a series of gradually diminishing cycles. Just as the body suffers a gradual decrease of vitality as it adjusts to destructive practices, it also experiences a gradual gain in vitality as we discontinue destructive living patterns.

For example, after starting on an improved diet you may feel much better for awhile. Sometimes, however, symptoms may occur—like headaches, nausea or diarrhea—after which you feel much better than before, and all goes well for a period of time thereafter.

Then a cold may come on with chills, fever, and loss of appetite. After a few days of rest, recovery comes and you feel better than ever. Then after a few months a skin rash develops and flares for a week and suddenly subsides (provided no drugs are taken and its allowed to run its course). Immediately after, you may find your energy levels increase dramatically.

Gradually, once the body reaches a reasonably high state of health, symptoms of detoxification that accompany the disease/healing process disappear or become minimal and the body remains in such a high state of health that very little discomfort is experienced during the body's stepped-up cleansing cycles.

And so it goes, each sensation milder than the last as the body becomes progressively purer. Each healing crisis is shorter in duration until a plateau of vibrant health is reached, and a bona fide state of permanent health is experienced.

A relatively disease-free state is then achieved and an acute clarity of mind which can only be attained by aligning ourselves with our biological requisites. Eat simple, pure, and natural foods properly prepared and combined, and the body will reap the benefits as we forsake destructive modes of eating and living.

Increasing our health also increases body awareness—the purer the body, the more aware you become of influences and substances that are harmful to your health and well-being, and we naturally become more sensitized to the body's needs. As major aches and pains disappear, minor irritations not previously noticed now enter our awareness. This represents an improvement in condition that guides us away from poor foods, unhealthful practices, and other life destroying habits.

Modern man has generally become desensitized and removed from the natural needs of his own body. Most people today have such a low level of body awareness that they do not realize that they are suffering from poor health until a severe blow lays them low.

A lack of body awareness accompanies a sickened condition—it is this very absence of "being in tune" with the body that permits the physiology to degenerate. As we become attuned to our biological needs, we become more aware that something is wrong in the lifestyle, which then can be adjusted (such as diet, fasting, etc.).

Most Food Consumed Is Not Suited to Our Physiology

All transgressions of our natural diet have pathological results whether evident or not. Man's physiology allows him to eat almost anything that does not immediately kill him.

It is a fatal mistake, however, to assume that the body can digest and assimilate everything that we masticate while entertaining our taste buds, or that foods which appear to do no *immediate* harm do not eventually cause problems. Consequently, most of what we eat is for naught, as most "food" consumed is, by and large, unsuited to the body's physiology.

The human body can be minimally maintained on an assortment of various foods—otherwise, our race would have long since become extinct. But like a gasoline engine that can operate on kerosene, it clogs up, parts wear out sooner, and its serviceable life is greatly reduced.

Similarly, the human body works best and lasts longest in a state of health when fed fuel on which it is intended to function optimally—a diet predominating in fresh raw fruits, vegetables, unsalted raw nuts and seeds, and sprouted grains and legumes. Our biological equipment is such that the body obtains complete and maximum nutrition without stress from plant foods and best survives accordingly.

When the body is abused by our modern traditional diet, the colon suffers the most as indicated by the high incidence of colon cancer. After several years on a conventional low-fiber diet, the average adult carries about 10-20 pounds of fecal matter on the colon walls. In many cases, the distended abdomens of those who are overweight are not due solely to fat as they are to the accumulation of feces over a period of years. Autopsies have revealed over 50 pounds of fecal material within some bodies.

When waste material moves slowly through the colon due to the intestinal wall becoming clogged and narrowed, or due to peristaltic nerves being paralyzed by toxicity from decaying foodstuffs, excessive water is reabsorbed and the feces harden, causing constipation. Fortunately, a diet high in NATURAL fiber from whole raw fruits and vegetables can greatly aid the body in restoring the health of the intestines.

The BEST source of dietary fiber is whole foods. Fragmented foods, such as bran, cause more problems since they cut, tear, and cause stress within the intestine and are not readily accepted by the body (bran may also cause loss of vital mineral elements). Their action is similar to a laxative, ultimately resulting in eventual inhibition of the body's ability to defecate for itself without being continually prodded and goaded to action.

The quality of our body largely depends upon the quality of food we eat, proper food combining, and the quantity consumed. Body chemistry is also influenced by the food we ingest.

When diet is altered and maintained, digestive enzymes, glandular secretions, and body fluids become increasingly adapted to the requirements of the new food program. Similarly, the body struggles to adapt when bombarded with junk food. The important difference is that adaptation to the misguided food program involves health deterioration, while re-adjustment in the direction of a more ideal food program is always towards improved health.

Junk foods are those that have been so altered and nutritionally impaired during processing, manufacturing, bleaching, canning, cooking and preserving that they no longer are suitable to meet the needs of the body as they were in their whole state as found in nature.

The body responds to all dietary influences and deals with them as they arise to best of its residual ability. When we consume food which is laden with contaminants such as artificial preservatives and additives, the body correctly treats these as poisons and attempts to eliminate them as rapidly as possible.

Those substances which cannot be removed through regular channels of elimination are stored in the body's vital and fatty tissues where they accumulate.

This forms the basis of a toxemic state, and the body eventually makes a concerted effort to rid itself of this unwanted debris—either in the form of a cold, flu, bronchitis, skin rash, diarrhea, or vomiting, etc. If the symptoms are suppressed, the basis of chronic disease is established.

Give the human body only those elements to which it is ideally adapted and it will provide pleasure and joy to its occupant. *Give the body junk foods, manufactured foods, denatured, and devitalized foods, drugs and insalubrious influences and it becomes clogged, impaired, and diseased.* If its needs are not adequately met, and if its functions are interrupted, the body cannot maintain normal, high levels of health and well-being.

Food should serve one primary purpose—to supply the body with materials it needs to maintain health. Junk foods CANNOT serve this function. Rather, they do just the opposite. Usable nutrients are denied to the body since sodas, cakes, chips, etc., cannot provide suitable materials required to generate healthy normal cells and in addition, are often nutrient antagonists.

Without the minimum necessary nutrients, the powers of life wane and poisons wreak havoc in the body. The number one child killer in this country is cancer, and this is why.

Over-nutrition and overeating are also harmful. The body's metabolic system can be likened to a funnel. Only a certain amount of food can pass through the funnel's small end, corresponding to the body's interior where only limited amounts of food can be "burned" efficiently to form energy, carbon dioxide, and water.

Also, the body's eliminative organs (intestines, liver, kidneys, lungs, and skin) can only eliminate a limited amount of excess foods. When too much food is poured into the funnel, a backup occurs. The bloodstream, intercellular spaces, and then our cells become overloaded with excess nutritive material and unremoved metabolic waste. Toxemia then develops.

A high caloric intake produces a toxic body that is unable to use energy efficiently. Waste clogs the body, impairs normal metabolic function, and demands high blood pressure for circulation.

The more food ingested, the more must be eliminated. When more is eaten than the body can utilize, a great deal of energy is wasted in converting and expelling the surplus.

Conservation of energy is the key to health and disease—we must eat enough biologically correct foods to supply the body with required nutrients but not so much that there is a surplus where excessive vital energy is expended in disposing of the overload.

Over-nutrition dissipates our energies and enervates the system. The result is inadequate nutrition, damage to the organism, disease, and premature aging.

The smallest amount of food able to keep the body in a state of high efficiency is physiologically the most economical, and is the best adapted diet for the body's needs. As health increases, the body's need for food *decreases* because of increased physiological efficiency, and weight maintenance and increased energy occurs with less food ingested.

Two meals a day easily becomes the norm for some, and for others, even one meal per day. The body not only becomes more efficient metabolically, but it also decreases in tissue breakdown during exercise and physical exertion. Less food is required to maintain a high quality of life.

The higher percentage of raw food we eat, the slower the rate of tissue degeneration. A sick body requires a gradual and carefully implemented entry into this stage, until the point at which one can thrive on a nearly 100% raw (unfired) diet.

The Role of Various Foods in Health and Disease

The human body must continuously deal with many different substances in the bloodstream, each of which has a range of concentration that can vary within certain limits without creating an imbalance of normal bodily functions. Blood glucose can vary up to 200% whereas blood calcium is constricted to a much narrower range of deviation.

The body maintains a proper pH balance at all times because it MUST do so in order for proper metabolic functioning to continue—the organism is designed that way.

To make this physiological function easier, and to conserve energy and vital alkaline mineral reserves, the diet should consist of foods that have an appropriate acid-alkaline ratio of at least 75% alkaline foods (which include fresh, raw fruits and vegetables), and not more than 25% acid foods (raw nuts and seeds).

If the diet is overloaded with acidic foods and/or foods deficient in base minerals (including refined, fragmented foods, junk foods, most grains and legumes, and meat and animal products), the body taps its base mineral reserves and literally robs the teeth and bones of calcium.

Examples of the body tapping its base mineral reserves include the consumption of white sugar; white flour; acid neutralization (as in uric acid from meat); or when the circulation's alkaline mineral supply is exhausted due to an overly acidic diet that is sparse in alkaline minerals. If continued for years, degenerative disease is the result, including osteoporosis, dental caries diabetes, hypoglycemia, nervousness, and depression.

When we refer to "alkaline foods," we mean food that leaves an alkaline "ash" residue after being metabolized, namely fresh fruits and vegetables. The alkaline properties of raw vegetables and nut proteins help maintain the body's acid-alkaline balance.

This is why the diet should consist of AT LEAST 75% alkaline-reacting foods and 25% or less acid-forming foods. (Most foods with high-protein content are acidic). Adherence to a varied Hygienic dietary along with vigorous regular exercise and other principles of Hygiene enables the body to adequately monitor its acid-alkaline balance and maintain pH equilibrium.

Ingestion of animal foods results in many acid by-products—most notably uric acid, sulfuric acid, and phosphoric acid, which cause the body's buffer systems (those organ's including the lungs and kidneys that maintain normal pH) to overwork and become enervated and eventually diseased.

It is these acid by-products of animal foods that tend to leach the tissues of their alkaline mineral salts which are needed, particularly by the body's cells, to buffer and render metabolic end-products less acidic and less irritating to the cells and tissues.

Since the average American diet is too high in protein, adding fruit to the diet is beneficial. Fruit burdens the digestion much less than other foods, freeing up energy which allows the body to accelerate its own "cleansing."

Fruits are mistakenly called "cleansing foods." Fruits do not of themselves cleanse the body, rather the body metabolically handles fruits so efficiently during digestion that it redirects much of the energy previously expended on biologically improper foods to the tasks of extraordinary elimination.

Sweet juicy fruits are so easily digested and replete with energy (glucose) that the body expends very little energy in their digestion, thereby reserving energy and resource for other physical processes such as cleansing, healing and repair. In addition, fresh fruit and their juices do not leave any toxic res-idues that the body has to contend with.

The human body metabolizes most acids in fruit very well. Benzoic acid, tannic acid, oxalic acid, and prussic acid are among those acids which give humans metabolic problems. (These are rare in fruits). The primary fruit acids are handled very well in our body—these include citric acid, malic acid, and tartartic acid.

When fruit acids DO occasion digestive problems it is because the acid fruit (lemons, limes, pineapple, strawberries, grapefruit, etc.) are either eaten for dessert when the stomach is already full; when the acid foods are combined improperly with sweet or dried fruit (like bananas, dates, figs, raisins, persimmons, etc.); when the acid fruit is spoiled or not ripened properly; or when fruit is cooked.

Overly cooked foods literally wreck our body. They deny needed nutrients to the system since heat alters foodstuffs such that they are partially, mostly, or wholly destroyed. Nutrients are coagulated, deaminized, caramelized and rendered inorganic and become toxic and pathogenic in the body.

Condiments and stimulants also vitiate our intestinal tract. Excess salt, herbs, spices, pepper, vinegar, dressings, sauces, seasonings, gravies, etc., all destroy our health.

Similarly, when spoiled or fermented food is eaten, the body rushes it to the nearest exit in an effort to protect itself. Sauerkraut, yogurt, pickles, etc., are hurried through the digestive tract where they are quickly expelled so as not to disrupt the body.

Fermented foods are NOT digested, but ARE quickly eliminated. If the food is extremely fermentative or putrefactive, diarrhea may occur as increased intestinal motility takes place as the body attempts to speedily eliminate the sub-standard food.

Proper fluid intake is also essential for the body's health.

The human body is about 70% water. The average person has about 45 quarts of fluid in his or her body at all times. Water is responsible for and involved in nearly every life process. During digestion, absorption, circulation, and excretion, water is the body's primary transporter of nutrients.

Water also helps maintain body temperature—on the average, about three quarts of water are lost each day in the form of perspiration, excretion, etc. This water must be replaced. Generally, three to four days is the longest the body can go without replacing these fluids before serious damage and eventual death occurs. Unfortunately, we tend to replace these fluids in ways that are harmful.

Pure water (distilled) is the only fluid which is used by the body. All other beverages must be regarded either as food or poison. Alcohol, caffeine, soft drinks, hot and cold beverages all contribute to poor health. (Alcohol actually *dehydrates* the body and causes fluids to be lost from the system).

The inside of the body is much more sensitive than its exterior. Hot drinks, cold drinks, irritating condiments, etc., destroy sensitive nerve endings, and disrupt body homeostasis and digestion.

As long as foods are eaten which are water sufficient—composed of 80-95% water, thirst will not occur and all of our water needs will be met in a biologically superior manner. (Almost all fresh succulent fruits and vegetables contain 80-95% pure water).

The only safe and correct diet for humans is one that meets all of the body's nutritional needs in a rational, satisfying manner without threat or stress to the system. The Hygienic food program does just that. Eat and live Hygienically, and your body will reach its highest potential for health and well-being and will serve you well throughout its entire life span.

SECTION V

BUT HOW ABOUT BACTERIA, GERMS, AND VIRUSES— AREN'T THEY THE CAUSE OF DISEASE?

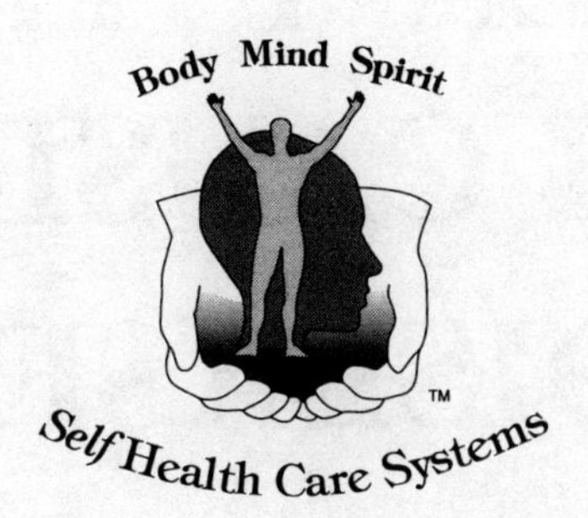
Body Mind Spirit
™
Self Health Care Systems

Chapter 14

FIRST SOME HISTORY: PASTEUR'S GERM THEORY OF DISEASE CAUSATION

In 1864, French chemist Louis Pasteur fathered *"The Science of Bacteriology"* and *"The Germ Theory of Disease Causation"* by demonstrating the existence of various microorganisms—and concluding that these germs cause pathogenic changes in living cultures within the laboratory setting.

The germ theory states that diseases are due solely to invasion by specific aggressive microorganisms. A specific germ is responsible for each disease, and microorganisms are capable of reproduction and transportation outside of the body.

With the germ theory of disease, no longer did we have to take responsibility for sickness caused by our own transgressions of the laws of health. Instead we blamed germs that invaded the body.

The germ theory effectively shifted our personal responsibility for health and well-being onto the shoulders of the medical profession who supposedly knew how to kill off the offending germs. Our own personal health slipped from our control.

Almost everyone in the Western world has been nurtured on the germ theory of disease—that disease is the direct consequence of the work of some outside agent, be it germ or virus.

People have been educated to be terrified of bacteria and to believe implicitly in the idea of contagion—that specific malevolently aggressive disease germs pass from one host to another. They also have been programmed to believe that healing requires some powerful force to remove whatever is at fault. In their view, illness is hardly their own doing.

The "germ-era" helped usher in the decline of hygienic health reform in the 19th century and, ironically, the people also found a soothing complacency in placing the blame for their ill health on malevolent, microscopic "invaders," rather than facing responsibility for their own insalubrious lifestyle habits and their own suffering.

Pasteur was a chemist and physicist and knew very little about biological processes. He *was* a respected, influential, and charismatic man, however, whose phobic fear of infection and belief in the "malignancy and belligerence" of germs had popular far-reaching consequences in the scientific community, which was convinced of the threat of the microbe to man. Thus, was born the fear of germs (bacteriophobia) which still exists today.

Before the discoveries of Pasteur, medical science was a

disorganized medley of diversified diseases with imaginary causes, each treated symptomatically rather than at their root cause. Up to this time, the evolution of medical thought had its roots in ancient shamanism, superstition, and religion—of invading entities and spirits. The profession searched in vain for a tangible basis on which to base its theories and practices. Pasteur then gave the profession the "germ."

By the 1870s, the medical profession fully adopted the germ theory with a vengeance that continues today. The advent of the microscope made it possible to see, differentiate, and categorize the organisms. Invading microbes were now seen as the cause of disease.

The medical-pharmaceutical industry began their relentless search for the perfect drug to combat each disease causing microbe—of which there are now over 10,000 distinct diseases recognized by the American Medical Association .

The universal acceptance of the germ theory and widespread bacteriophobia resulted in frenzied efforts to avoid the threat of germs. A whole new era of modern medicine was then inaugurated including sterilization, pasteurization, vaccination, and fear of eating raw food.

Medical authorities advised the public to cook all food thoroughly and to boil water. With the deprivation of raw foods, an inevitable deterioration of health ensued.

The practice of killing germs with drugs was also initiated, resulting in iatrogenic (medically-induced) disease and further degeneration of health. Various programs were instituted to confer "immunity" against specific germs by way of vaccines and serums, with horrendous effects.

Fortunately, the horror of consuming raw food as being dangerous and bacteria ridden has largely been overcome, although the ban on unpasteurized dairy foods still exists in most of this country. And the acceptance of poisonous drugs and inoculations has not waned to any appreciable extent.

Scientific Contradictions to Pasteur's Germ Theory—Koch's Four Postulates

Scientists in the medical field pose as being bound by *postulates* —which are self-evident axioms, statements or prepositions that bear out inherent evidence of their truth. Robert Koch, the German pioneer of microbiology, derived a series of criteria that should be met in the laboratory to establish the causal relationship between an organism and a disease supposedly associated with it.

Robert Koch (1843-1910) was a contemporary of Louis Pasteur. He formulated four postulates which maintained that for a specific bacteria to be the cause of a disease:

1. It must be found in every case of that disease;
2. It must **not** be found when the disease is **not** present;
3. It must be capable of living outside the tissues; and
4. It must then be capable of re-introduction into the organism and produce that disease.

The first two of Koch's postulates state that if a disease is caused by a certain bacterium, then that bacterial strain must always be present when the disease exists. The other postulates state that the particular disease must always be occasioned by the presence or introduction of the bacteria said to be responsible.

In other words, Koch's postulates say that the suspected microorganism has to be present in all cases of the disease it is said to cause. In addition, the microorganism must be able to be taken from an infected host, animal or human and further spread in a laboratory culture.

Finally, Koch's postulates state that inoculations of the microorganism into unaffected animals must produce in them the original disease and the bacteria or infecting agent must be found present in the experimental host so infected. In short, the presence of the causative agency must always occasion the same illness.

Koch negated Pasteur's original germ theory by presenting his four postulates in 1892. *Although these cardinal principles are self-evident, so many exceptions exist as to totally disprove the germ theory of disease causation—and the medical profession has never given them credence* .

By 1900 it was scientifically evident that the germ theory of disease would not stand-up, as it had repeatedly been demonstrated that specific bacteria do not fulfill these prerequisites to be considered causative factors in disease.

Koch's postulates destroyed the theory even though vestiges of the concept still survive today (as in strep throat). In the early part of this century as pharmaceutical interests took over medical educational institutions, bacterial culprits were slowly replaced with "viruses."

"Susceptibility" vs. Actual Causality

Relative to modern medical theory, Koch's postulates are a modification of the germ theory, requiring the condition of SUSCEPTIBILITY to establish a bona fide causal relationship between specific germs and specific diseases.

Today, the word "susceptible" has been fraudulently interpolated into Koch's postulates by the medical establishment. When the condition of SUSCEPTIBILITY is introduced, the situation radically changes, as *the condition of the host is then of primary importance in the production of disease.*

The word "susceptible" means that the criterion which establishes susceptibility is the actual cause of disease and not the microorganism or the agency blamed.

Anyone who quotes the postulates with the word "susceptible" in them is not quoting Koch—the word has been added to explain away the fact that experimental hosts rarely develop the disease that the blamed infective agent is supposed to cause.

Unless a germ will cause a disease every time it "infects" the body, it is not a cause. A cause must be consistent and specific in its influence or it is not a cause. Germs are omnipresent and yet fail to have a specific influence all the time.

Scientists know that specific bacteria are not always found in each case of the disease they are supposedly responsible for. In 28-40% of diphtheria cases, diphtheria bacillus is absent. Koch's first postulate "the specific bacteria must be found in every case of that disease" is not fulfilled in diphtheria, tuberculosis, typhoid fever, pneumonia, OR ANY OTHER DISEASE.

Nor is the second postulate fulfilled since it is a medically known fact that bacteria are routinely found in the bodies of animals and humans who exhibit NO symptoms of *any* disease. Neither is the third postulate satisfied since virulent "disease germs" are dependent on human or animal organisms for their survival and are not capable of surviving outside the tissues. And finally, neither is Koch's fourth postulate fulfilled.

Quoting from the article *"The Germ Theory Reexamined"* by Bob Zuraw and Bob Lewanski (in the September-November 1977 edition of *Vegetarian World*): "Koch's Fourth Postulate, namely, introducing germ cultures in a healthy body or organism, DOES NOT produce signs and symptoms of disease."

"The Bio-Chemical Society of Toronto conducted a number of experiments where pure cultures of meningitis, typhoid, diphtheria, pneumonia, and tuberculosis germs were consumed by the millions in food and drink by volunteers. No ill effects resulted whatsoever."

According to Dr. Herbert Shelton, germs alone could no

more cause disease than a match alone can produce a fire. If the microbe is to have any part in causing disease it must find an organism that produces suitable soil for its metabolic activities. We cannot avoid germs—they are everywhere—we must be proof against them. We avoid disease, then, only by keeping ourselves in such a state of health that germs are powerless against us.

Pasteur Not the Originator of the "Germ Theory"

Actually, the first "Germ Theory of Infectious Disease" was published in 1762 (almost 100 years prior to Pasteur's theory) by a Viennese physician Dr. M.A. Plenciz. In 1860, Louis Pasteur took the credit for the experiments and theory and became identified as its originator. Read the books "Pasteur: Plagiarist, Imposter" by R.B. Pearson, and "Be'champ or Pasteur? A Lost Chapter in the History of Biology." by Douglas E. Hume for all the details.

Claude Bernard (1813-1878) disputed the validity of the germ theory and maintained that **the general condition of the body is the principal factor in disease**, but this idea was largely ignored by the medical profession and the general public. Bernard and Pasteur had many debates on the relative importance of the microbe and the internal environment in which they thrive.

Pasteur Realizes Mistake

Around 1880, Pasteur himself admitted his mistake. According to Dr. Duclaux (one of Pasteur's co-workers), Pasteur discovered that microbial species can undergo many transformations. These facts were not consistent with his germ theory and destroyed its very basis.

It is frequently overlooked that around 1880, Pasteur changed his theory. According to Dr. Duclaux, Pasteur stated that germs were "ordinarily kept within bounds by natural laws but when conditions change, when its virulence is exalted, when its host is enfeebled, the germ is able to invade the territory which was previously barred to it.". This is the premise that a healthy body is resistant and not susceptible to disease.

With the advent of Pasteur's mysterious germ, however, medicine cloaked itself under the guise of "science" and ever since has succeeded in keeping the public ignorant of the true nature of disease.

Chapter 15

BACTERIA AND THEIR SYMBIOTIC ROLE IN THE BODY

Bacteria are living entities called *eukaryotes* or *prokaryotes* . Bacteria are our symbiotic partners in life and are completely normal to the body. They work symbiotically with the host organism by assisting in the breakdown and removal of toxic materials and in creating nutrients that are vital to our welfare.

Lactobacillus acidophilus , *lactobacillus bifidus* , and *coli* bacteria are normally present in the human digestive tract and are sometimes called "friendly, beneficial, or symbiotic intestinal flora." They are necessary within the body for the proper absorption and utilization of food particles; for aiding in cellular nourishment; for stimulating peristalsis; for detoxifying and creating soft, smooth stools; and for keeping down pathogenic germs. (Antibiotics destroy these forms of useful bacteria).

Bacteria and microorganisms also form a vital part in the world's food chain. When organic matter within plants and animals decompose throughout nature, bacteria and molds of the *Monera* family disorganize the highly complex organic molecules into simple inorganic wastes whose elements are excreted back into the soil to be taken up once again as food by plants, and reorganized via the process of photosynthesis into widely diverse forms of vegetable matter, including food for humans such as fruits, nuts, and seeds.

Bacteria are actually a primitive form of life, which subsist on scavenging dead organic material. They break-up and decompose waste material in our system, just as they do within the plant and animal kingdoms.

Bacterial action renders some waste matters usable in our body that would ordinarily be expelled and, as such, bacteria are essential to our lives—without them our existence would not be possible. As intestinal flora, for instance, bacteria are a much needed symbiotic partner in life, responsible for synthesizing vitamin B-12 and vitamin K within our body.

Our body carries about a five year supply of vitamin B-12, and receives a constantly refurnished supply from bacterial activity in the lower intestine, just as is the case with other primates and natural plant-eating animals, **including man**. Also, vitamin K does not need to be supplied by food since bacteria which live symbiotically in the human intestine are capable of producing this nutrient, which is required for normal functioning of the body's bloodclotting agents.

The Beneficial Role of Bacteria in Disease

As a cause of disease, bacteria do not "invade" the body—for they are already present in the digestive tract (which, by the way, technically IS considered outside the body proper). As needed, bacteria are brought into the circulatory system to aid in the process of purging the physiology of accumulated wastes.

When the body creates a highly localized toxic condition in the system, as occurs during inflammation, the body absorbs bacteria from the intestines and/or other body cavities and transports them to where the accumulated poisons have been concentrated.

During the inflammatory process, pus is formed from the aggregate of dead cells and from the healing white blood cell activity that takes place, and bacteria proliferate to feast on and process this material which makes it easier for the body to expel.

In this way, bacteria symbiotically assist in breaking down these toxic materials for elimination. In the process however, the excreta of bacteria generated therein is toxic. The bacteria's own excretion reflects the morbidity of the toxins they consume in that these wastes are also highly virulent. If not eliminated from the body, these accumulate to such an extent that the body initiates a cleansing/healing crisis.

Bacteria do not produce disease but are useful organisms that help decompose dead cellular material when the body's cells have completed their normal life cycle.

This process helps eliminate the dead matter from the body and, likewise, the bacteria aid in clearing toxic substances. This is why they are seen regularly during the disease/purification process since these processes require the disintegration of accumulated poisonous refuse which the system is endeavor-ingto purge.

Bacteria do not cause the death of the organic matter on which they act, however, as they are a part of the RESULT of disease, NOT ITS CAUSE.

Bacteria and germs play an important role in the evolution of disease but are not fundamental causes as commonly believed. Bacteria are intimately associated with serious illness, but merely contribute secondary or tertiary complicating factors by elaborating certain powerful toxins already present in the toxic body due to the poisonous by-products of their own fermentative and putrefactive actions.

Lactic acid, acetic acid (vinegar), alcohol from the fermentation process; and ammonias, indoles, skatols and purines, etc., from the putrefaction process are toxic—although our body under normal conditions of health can easily eliminate these forms of bacterial excreta. In fact, our feces and urine are loaded with these protein decomposition by-products both from bacterial activity and our own body metabolism.

Bacteria need nourishment to grow and reproduce. When there is a dangerous accumulation of waste materials which is threatening body integrity, our symbiotic bacteria go into action and perform their janitorial/scavenging function of clearing the body of filth and debris. Afterwards, they resume their passive state once again.

Bacteria have an important role to perform in the vital process of healing. Germs take part in virtually all disease phenomena that require the disintegration of refuse and toxic matter within the body which the system is endeavoring to remove. They act as scavengers in clearing up the affected area of toxic saturation. As soon as their role is complete, their numbers decline.

For this reason once again, bacteria are associated with

disease processes BUT ARE NOT ITS CAUSE, for bacteria no more cause disease than flies cause garbage. To assume that because germs are present and active in the decomposition processes connected with dead organic matter, that they cause its death is erroneous.

When toxicosis exists and threatens the well-being of the organism, the body responds by purging the toxins, and disease symptoms appear. Bacteria are present to decompose metabolic wastes, toxins, dead cells ad tissues and, as such, are a vitally important part of the healing process.

Bacteria are capable of only one action in regard to the disease process: the processing of dead materials as their food. Bacteria proliferate because there is dead organic matter for them to feed on, not because they suddenly become malevolent.

In a relatively sterile environment, they die due to lack of nourishment just as they similarly die off in an environment of their own creating—namely, in the presence of their own toxic excreta including lactic acid, acetic acid, alcohol, ammonia and numerous other protein decomposition by-products.

It is inappropriate to call bacterial activity an "attack" or an "invasion" on the part of germs, unless we mean it is an attack on the toxins. The only real attack that takes place, is the one WE make upon our own body as we continually assault ourselves on the average of some 30 poisoning acts each day—including the devitalized "foods" and "beverages" we consume, the drugs we take, constantly staying up late, and overeating needlessly, all of which create enervation and exhaustion of the body.

On the other hand, bacteria *cannot* thrive in healthy blood. This is why a clean, well-nourished body is not subject to their presence.

Living in a germ-free environment is impossible, however, and not even wholly desirable. Trillions of bacteria live in our body at all times. If we were free of them we would soon die since they aid in digestion and actually generate vitamins for the body. Provided we keep our internal and external environment clean, germs and bacteria serve a useful purpose.

Bacteria Mutate According to Decomposing Soil in the Environment

There are no "disease producing" bacteria, germs, microbes, bacilli, or viruses—it is the environment and the host which determine disease symptoms and the type of bacteria that proliferate. **Germs do not cause disease, rather *the body generated disease* occasions the germ proliferation that takes place.**

In order for a particular germ to exist, it has to have a suitable environment created by the toxic and pathological pollution saturating the body. Systemic poisoning then creates the specific germ culture, depending upon where the body has accumulated the wastes and according to the unhealthful lifestyle habits of the sufferer.

The key point is, however, that it is the diseased toxemic condition, where the body is overwhelmed with poisonous waste, which creates an environment favorable to the *mutation* of bacteria into those commonly associated with particular diseases. The disease condition favors proliferation and increasing virulence until their function of devouring toxic debris is accomplished.

When you ask a bacteriologist what comes first, the soil or the bacteria, the answer is always the tainted environment, in order for the bacteria to thrive. Bacteria never exist in a proliferating state where there is no food or soil for their propagation—but they multiply rapidly when there is decomposing material to feast on, and then they die off when there is famine or adversity in their surroundings.

Once again, bacteria no more create their food supply than flies cause garbage. The garbage or soiled state within our body must pre-exist the presence of bacterial "invasion"—**bacteria do not cause disease, they are present because of it.**

Bacteriologists themselves wrongly divide the germ population into specific "good germs" and "bad germs" and overlook the fact that "good germs" have the ability to mutate and proliferate into "bad" virulent germs when their soil is suitable for this change.

In other words, germs can modify their structure and metabolic function according to the environment in which they find themselves. They exist in a multitude of strains, shapes, and metabolic capabilities and may appear as rod-shaped or circular shaped depending on the dictates of their environment.

The germ theory was founded on the assumption that disease germs are specific, unchangeable entities in their biological structure and chemical characteristics. The 1968 Pulitzer Prize winner and eminent bacteriologist Dr. Rene J. Dubos contradicted this assumption, showing that the virulence of microbial species is variable.

As far back as 1914 in the *Journal of Infectious Diseases*, experiments by E.C. Risenow M.D. of the Mayo Biological Laboratories in Rochester, Minnesota demonstrated that pus germs (streptococci) can be transformed into pneumonia germs (pneumococci) simply by making minor alterations in their environment and by feeding them on pneumonia virus—dead organic matter characteristic with the manifestation of the disease.

When the procedure is reversed, the bacteria quickly revert back to the pus germs. In each case when the environment and food source were changed, the germs regardless of type quickly mutated into other forms.

Two New York City bacteriologists in similar experiments, converted cocci (round, berry-shaped bacteria) into bacilli (long, rod-shaped bacteria) and back again. A coccus (pneumonia germ) can change to a bacillus (typhoid germ) simply by making minor alterations in its environment and by feeding it typhoid virus—specific dead organic matter which is particular to this type of bacteria proliferation.

When the procedure is reversed, typhoid germs revert to pneumonia germs illustrating that, indeed, any bacteria can modify and adapt its structure and metabolic function in accordance with its changing environment. The virulence of germs can likewise be altered in the laboratory at will by the technician.

The Toxic Body Produces the Virulent Germ

It is evident, then, that germs do not directly produce disease—rather the body generated healing crisis produces the germ by providing a suitable environment where non-toxic bacteria mutate into toxic microorganisms within septic surroundings. For germs to become dangerous they must be intermingled with concentrated waste products before the germ metamorphosizes into a toxic entity.

While it is true that germs and bacteria exist everywhere, the microorganisms ONLY proliferate in the body when a person develops toxemia as a result of an unhealthy lifestyle.

Particular bacteria cause particular diseases they are associated with about as much as flies cause garbage. Both are scavenger forms of life. No garbage, no flies—likewise, no organic body exudates in the throat, lungs, respiratory tract, or elsewhere, no virulent bacteria to speak of.

When high quantities of oxidized organic material are being extraordinarily eliminated by the body via the throat, lungs or elsewhere, bacteria multiply geometrically. In hours, they may number in the trillions but suitable "soil" must be present before they can proliferate.

Strep throat and sore throat are said to be caused by streptococcus bacteria. This is a common form of bacteria in the lactobacilli family, a round-shaped organism that also breaks down or sours milk.

You can easily prepare a culture containing billions of strep bacteria as in yogurt, and any healthy person eating the yogurt will not develop strep throat. Put them in a milk culture and in hours they multiply into trillions. It is difficult to find anyone who does not contain this form of bacteria in their throat except in those using massive amounts of antibiotics or other life destroying drugs.

Streptococci are not in themselves dangerous, however, for millions of them are found in the average person's throat and body cavities—but their excrement can be highly toxic as they help breakdown, decompose, and putrefy waste materials which the body then eliminates through the lungs, throat, mucous membranes, and/or skin.

A sore throat is actually an irritation of the tissues, caused either by what is being eliminated there or by some injurious substance sent down it. Streptococcus bacteria use the exudates as soil. When a concentration of toxic material is available, their reproduction is tremendous. To reiterate however, streptococci are not harmful bacteria as they are always a normal portion of the body's flora.

Scientists know that specific bacteria are not always found in each case of the disease they are supposed to cause. Introducing germ cultures in a healthy body does not consistently generate disease symptoms. Numerous experiments feeding pure cultures of typhoid, pneumonia, diphtheria, tuberculosis, and meningitis germs produced no ill effects.

As mentioned before, in 28-40% of diphtheria cases, diphtheria bacillus is absent. Likewise, in about 20% of those suffering venereal disease (syphilis, herpes, gonorrhea, etc.) neither gonococcus nor spirochetes are present. Saying that bacteria causes an ulcer, pustule, or pimple about the genitals disregards the fact that these result from the body's autolysis (self-digestion) of tissue. The creation of boils and inflammations characteristic of V.D. are vital body actions, not bacterial or viral invasions.

Similarly, pneumonia is thought to be caused by the bacterium pneumococcus, although it is absent in more than a 25% of cases. Moreover, administering the bacterium to healthy organisms does not occasion the disease.

Even during the early stages of the common cold, nasal secretions are completely void of bacteria as none are found in the thin watery mucus in the first two to three days. When thick purulent secretion begins, pneumococci, staphlococci, and streptococci appear. Since bacteria are so conspicuously absent at the onset of a cold, another cause had to be found. Now, 150 different viruses are blamed for the affliction.

Colds are not "caught," rather they develop from our enervating way of life. Bacteria or viruses have nothing to do with the development of colds. They may be complicating features, since bacteria function as saprophytes (scavengers) feeding on the debris being eliminated. As long as tissues remain abnormal, bacteria thrive. Once the eliminative and purging actions are completed, they subside.

Physicians readily admit that they do not know exactly which virus causes colds, for when the cold virus is sprayed into throats it causes inflammation in ***"susceptible hosts only"*** —in those whose tissues are already irritated by foreign agents. In addition, so-called respiratory pathogenic bacteria ARE present in throat washings of those who have colds, but killing the microorganisms DOES NOT shorten the period of illness.

Colds are preventable but first we must learn their

causes. As long as it is assumed that germs and viruses cause colds and that we "catch" them, and as long as our efforts are directed against these microscopic entities, the cold will prevail. Colds are actually remedial efforts made necessary by the accumulation in the blood, lymph, and tissues of unexcreted metabolic waste and by the intestinal absorption of toxic by-products of indigestion.

The ultimate causes of the cold are habits of living which reduce digestive efficiency, check elimination, and cause enervation, permitting the internal environment to become polluted—a state of physiological smog, if you will.

Unless a germ will cause a disease every time it "infects" the body, it is not a cause. A cause must be consistent and specific in its influence. Germs are omnipresent and fail to have a specific influence all the time.

Both laboratory evidence and empirical observations substantiate that disease is the body's reaction to intoxication, and not to germs—**bacteria do not invade nor control the body, for they are always within the physical domain.**

The Body Controls its Bacterial Population

Normal healthy organisms are actually deadly to germs and parasites and have innate, built in resources to handle them. Bacteria are helpless against living cells, especially white blood cells and others that compose our natural lines of defense.

We harbor countless billions of microorganisms within our intestinal tract, within our skin, in our mouth, nose, and other body cavities.

The celebrated Dr. Lewis Thomas, who heads the Sloan-Kettering Cancer Institute said "pity not the man who has caught bacteria, rather pity the bacteria that was caught by the man." Humans furnish a very rough environment for bacteria, keeping them tightly restricted and controlled.

Lymph nodes—the glandular tissue masses that occur along the lymphatic vessels throughout the body—routinely remove bacteria and foreign particles from the general lymph circulation and supply lymphocytes to the circulatory system. The lymph nodes and spleen form a portion of the body's *reticuloendothelial system* —referring to those phagocytic cells scattered throughout the body which can ingest bacteria, solid particles, and other errant cells. This aids in keeping the body in a healthy, stable condition.

For example, billions and even trillions of bacteria and fungi are incidentally absorbed from the intestinal tract into the portal blood each day. These are so effectively apprehended and destroyed by our white blood cells and macrophages that scarcely any bacteria or fungi ever enter the circulating blood.

Leukocytes (white corpuscles) are the blood's defensive organisms that prevent intoxication by bacteria, cooked food debris, or other toxic materials. Leukocytosis (an excessive proliferation of white blood cells in the circulation) occurs in response to inflammation, to excessive numbers of bacteria in the body, and to a preponderance of cooked food—all of which represent pathological phenomena.

The body must exist in a toxic state before it will institute the disease process. Neither bacteria nor anything else can start and sustain a healing crisis—microorganisms are incapable of unified action and cannot exist where there is no food (soil) for them to survive. Living healthy cells are not soil for bacteria, but decomposing substances are.

If a *healthy* body can "catch" a cold or flu due to influenza germs and is unable to resist an "attack" by these microorganisms, then how can the subsequently *debilitated* body ever recover? How can the weakened organism repel the onslaught of trillions of proliferating microorganisms? The inevitable result would be the death of the organism.

If bacteria did invade organisms and subsequently lay them low, as medically supposed, the impetus and momentum they build-up in the process would become progressively more pronounced and overwhelming as the organism recedes further into disease.

If germs and microbe "attackers" overwhelmed a healthy body, then once they laid a victim low their proliferating reproduction would exponentially increase the "devouring," which would cease only when they had exhausted their food supply—there would be no recovery. If bacteria and viruses cause disease and debilitate the body, how does the weakened individual recover?

Were germs the cause of disease, there would be no remission, and germ proliferation would continue unimpeded.

Once the invading entities have a head-start, it does not seem they would stop their destruction but, instead, would further diminish the organism's ability to defend itself. When bacteria start decomposing a body, only complete exhaustion of all organic materials ends their course—only when "the bones are picked clean" so to speak.

Logic tells us that if microbial organisms "make someone sick" and proliferate by the billions as they become more numerous and stronger, they would progressively sap more and more energy, vitality and resources from their victim. How can this process be reversed by a much weakened organism?

The whole concept of being laid low by micro-

bes and then turning the tables on them makes for good fiction, but is physiologically false. For once dominance is established in nature over a weakened organism, its downhill from there. Once zebras are overwhelmed by carnivores, they rarely survive. Once bacteria start decomposing organic matter, they continue until their food source is exhausted.

The body does not suppress the growth and multiplication of "disease germs" until the morbid toxins on which they subsist have been consumed, and until the inflammatory process has run its course.

When diseases are said to be "limited" by medical authorities this really means the illness is a body detoxification process that is terminated by the body when its purging objectives are reached. The body is in control, and not at the mercy of hordes of microbes or some "mysterious disease entity."

Disease once more, is not caused by germs but by the toxic state of the body which allows the germ to flourish. This deranged state of the organism is the outgrowth of violating our biological requirements, and is no chance or haphazard condition.

It is this diseased condition that creates an environment favorable to the mutation of bacteria into those associated with specific disease, and to their increasing virulence and proliferation.

A state of internal cleanliness, therefore, is essential for health and well-being. A pure bloodstream, free unimpeded circulation of all body fluids, and unobstructed excretion generate and maintain healthy tissue. Virulent bacteria soon die in this environment for want of suitable nourishment.

If the microbe is to have any part in causing disease it must find an organism that produces suitable soil for its metabolic activities. We cannot avoid germs for they are everywhere

—we must be proof against them. We avoid disease only by keeping ourselves in such a state of health that germs are powerless against us.

The Medical Rationale of "Susceptibility" and "Resistance"

Everyone has literally trillions of fungi, bacteria, and "viruses" in their body even when healthy. When physicians are confronted with this they say that disease is not caused by these agencies because you are not "susceptible" or because "your resistance is high."

This is a cop out, saying that these agents DO NOT cause disease, *but those factors which dispose us to susceptibility* ***DO*** —since the word "susceptible" means that the criterion which establishes susceptibility is the actual cause of disease, and not the microorganism or the agency blamed. *This cop out confirms that the supposed contagious agents—bacteria, viruses and fungi DO NOT cause disease.* ***The actual cause is whatever CAUSES susceptibility or low resistance.***

If we maintain our body in a clean, healthy state then germs are irrelevant, for "susceptibility" does not exist. The concept of "susceptibility" is really the medical rationale which admits that bacteria only proliferate when the internal physiological condition warrants it. To repeat, it is an admission that an unclean environment is really the cause of disease—for if germs were the cause of disease, everyone exposed to the harmful germ would become sick with the same illness.

When the condition of SUSCEPTIBILITY is introduced into medical theory to describe disease causation, ***the condition of the host is then of primary importance in the production of disease.***

"Susceptible" individuals are those with a high degree of

body toxicity AND sufficient vitality to conduct the disease/purification process. When such sufficient vitality is waning, organic tissue damage occurs from the extraordinarily polluted internal state of the body which creates the foundation for chronic disease. So long as our body is relatively pure, however, waste materials do not accumulate and the scavenging assistance of bacterial germs are not called upon.

Physicians say that our RESISTANCE against germs is our only protection to avoid disease, but they leave their patients ignorant of how to guarantee a high degree of RESISTANCE at all times. We are told that germs invade only when resistance is lost. But what causes a loss of resistance? Obviously, loss of health means diminished resistance.

So if health is the best protection against disease, why not promote health by educating the populous in the requisites of health according to their biological mandate? **WHY NOT CREATE A TRUE *"HEALTH CARE"* SYSTEM, INSTEAD OF THE PREVAILING *"DISEASE CARE"* SYSTEM that currently exists?** We must promote health by living life according to those factors upon which health is generated.

Avoid Virulent Bacteria By Eating Healthfully

If we live and eat healthfully, the microbes within us will remain beneficent and you will only appreciate good health. The "bad" (virulent) bacteria and fungi ARE with us all the time but normally in such small numbers that in those who live healthfully, the bacteria do not generate significant amounts of noxious material due to lack of nutriment.

Raw fooders who live on a biologically correct diet of mostly raw fruit, vegetables, nuts and seeds have almost a total lack of putrefactive bacteria in their intestines.

Bacteria and fungi do not survive on the living substances of raw foods—nutriment must first oxidize to become soil for microbes. Instead, they live on dead organic matter such as cooked foods or carcasses but are innocuous to healthy organisms.

The following dietary factors are instrumental in causing abnormal amounts of decaying soil within the body for bacteria to ferment and putrefy:

1. Biologically incorrect foods;
2. Incorrect food combining of carbohydrates with fats and/or proteins at the same meal;
3. Overeating;
4. Cooked foods—heat deranges nutrients and encourcourages decay;
5. Oils, condiments, salt, sauces, etc., which usually retard or suspend digestion altogether;
6. Beverages consumed with meals—they dilute digestive juices and interfere with enzymatic activity;
7. Insufficient mastication and inadequate insalivation; and
8. Eating fermented foods (vinegar, alcohol, sauerkraut, pickles, relish, yogurt, cheese, etc.) which all retard or suspend digestion.

The only time mold, germs, or bacteria within raw food could reproduce and cause problems in the digestive canal is when the intestines and stomach are already toxic. Bacteria then find a smorgasbord of food laid out before them and ideal conditions in which to multiply. They become fat and healthy, excreting their own toxic by-products which add to those already present within the body.

The only healthy way to rid the intestinal tract of these pests is to remove their food supply by undergoing a fast. When we fast, the digestive system is emptied and putrefactive bacteria therein are disposed of. In the healthy individual, microorganisms are digested just as any other proteinaceous substance.

As mentioned before, virulent bacteria find soil in dead food substances only and cannot exist on living cells. Cooked food spoils readily, both inside and outside our body, whereas living foods are slow to lose their vital qualities and do not as readily become soil for bacterial decay.

Take milk as an example. When making yogurt, if you take RAW milk and add a culture of bacillus bulgaricus, the culture dies before souring the milk. But if you first boil and pasteurize the milk (and render it dead), then cool it to 100-110 degrees and add bacterial culture, you will have yogurt in six to eight hours. Bacteria cannot act on fresh, raw milk but once dead, the milk readily becomes soil for bacterial proliferation.

Cooked starches and sugars also spoil and ferment quickly and the body becomes a vinegar and alcohol factory, a cesspool if you will. Indigestion occurs and most of the food is acted upon by bacteria and not by our digestive juices—as these are no longer secreted when the digestive tract is vitiated. *Instead, the digestive tract seeks to DIVEST, rather than digest.*

Some 20% of the ordinary person's fecal matter is dead bacteria and fungi. This unusually large amount of expired bacteria is only true, however, for those who subsist on conventionally cooked foodstuffs.

The average American has about two pounds of bacteria in the intestinal tract, whereas healthy raw fooders have only a few ounces. Why? Those living on a biologically correct diet have very little fermentation and virtually no putrefaction.

To understand this further, take two apples—cook one and set it beside the other in the raw state. At room temperature, the cooked apple will ferment within 24-36 hours whereas the raw apple keeps fresh for at least 24-36 days! Cooked foods within our intestinal tract at some 96 degrees plus, quickly ferment or putrefy depending upon their predominating nutrient composite.

Plaque is the acid waste by-product of bacterial colonies that live in our mouth. As bacteria eat, they excrete an acid substance that forms the chalky plaque which coats the teeth.

When fresh (one or two days old), plaque can be brushed or flossed off, but if left on the teeth for long, it mineralizes into a rock-hard substance called *calculus* which becomes razor sharp and destroys teeth and gums unless dentally removed.

In addition, cooked grains (especially refined) lead to rapid dental decay. Cooked grains are soft and sticky and remain on the teeth for bacteria to digest. Unless supplemented by high-calcium fresh leafy greens, grain meals lead to excessive phosphorus and acid levels in the body which cause cavities.

Cavities are not caused by bacterial formation of acids in the mouth as is commonly believed. Cavities are primarily caused by an improper diet.

Refined sugars, acid-forming foods, and high phosphorus foods are the true culprits. Sucrose and refined sugars cause osteoporosis of bones and teeth. The body is forced to borrow base minerals (especially calcium) from its reserves to metabolize sugar and neutralize acid radicals in order to maintain an alkaline pH of its blood and tissue fluids.

By eating a biologically correct diet cavities will not form. If the diet is substandard, even brushing and flossing the teeth are ineffective in preventing cavities as is drinking fluoridated water.

The rationale for adding inorganic fluorine into our tap water to supposably curb tooth decay is that the mineral is toxic to some of the bacteria residing in the mouth. Inorganic fluorine DOES NOT make tooth enamel harder and more resistant to tooth decay. Instead, inorganic fluorine displaces certain chemical ions in the enamel which makes it less soluble and results in the storage of the mineral.

Actually, fluorine does not prevent tooth decay one iota, since bacteria no more cause cavities than they cause any other disease. The fact that inorganic fluorine DOES kill bacteria should make you wary of the deadly substance, for this illustrates its poisonous character. In many areas of the world, people have excellent teeth without a trace of inorganic fluorine in the water supply.

Naturally occurring ORGANIC fluorine as found in small amounts within whole foods IS a beneficial mineral for the teeth, but the harsh inorganic form of fluorine that is commonly dumped into our water supply is actually a hazardous waste by-product from industrial manufacturing and fertilizer production.

Chemical and metal industries profitably unload their fluoride toxic pollutants into public drinking water in the name of dental hygiene. You cannot drink a chemical and expect to have healthy teeth—good teeth are built only through proper nutrition.

To reiterate, dental cavities ARE NOT created by the external action of acidic bacterial excretion on the surface of the teeth as is commonly thought, but by mineral imbalances created in the body by improper foods and beverages.

Animal flesh and its derivatives such as beef tea or bouillon are also perfect media for the multiplication of bacteria. When proteins have been cooked or preserved, enzymes are coagulated and their cleavage into component amino acids is inhibited and may not be liberated for synthesis into body structure. Instead they become soil for bacteria, and poisonous decomposition by-products are generated.

Protein which remains in the stomach for too long, permits the overdevelopment of harmful bacteria. The poisonous excreta from the bacteria coupled with the incompletely digested and decomposing proteins are absorbed directly into the bloodstream. **Man is not a true carnivore and cannot digest flesh protein properly, and putrefaction invariably results which contributes to the development of disease.**

Meat and flesh foods, once slaughtered, begin to decom pose rapidly. Bacteria thrive in this environment and, when eaten, parasitic infections can be transmitted to man. Outbreaks of staphylococcal enteritis, shigella dysentery, and salmonella are often traced to meat improperly preserved and/or prepared. Oysters and shellfish also cause infectious hepatitis when taken from contaminated water where human waste levels are high.

Parasitic infections are frequently traced to meat-based diets. Beef, pork, and fish containing tapeworms cause anemia, weakness, and chronic disability.

Consumer Reports (February 1972) studied samples from 32 brands of supermarket frankfurters throughout the U.S. Food experts agree that putrefaction has set in when frankfurter bacteria count has reached 10 million per gram. More than 40% of the samples analyzed had begun to spoil using this measuring scale. (One sample tested out at 140 million bacteria per gram).

In addition, results of a nationwide survey of pork revealed that "whether the sausage came from a federally-inspected meat packing plant or from a local butcher's meat grinder, it was often sour or rancid and frequently contaminated with an overabundance of bacteria and filth. Not one sample of the packages as tested for quality and flavor could be judged really outstanding."

Trinchinosis is the most rampant parasitic disease that is transported within meat, and the U.S. leads the world in incidence rates of trinchinosis—about three times as much as the rest of the world COMBINED.

Approximately 16% of all adults autopsied in this country are found to have trinchinosis, for which there is no cure. Heavy infections may cause death but, more often, the only symptoms of trichinosis are chronic aches and pains that are usually passed off as arthritis or rheumatism.

Properly cooked meat, poultry, and seafood kills the bacteria and parasites but when eaten raw (or after just a brief exposure to heat), one is inviting bacterial or parasitic disease. Avoid meat eating and avoid these parasitic infections.

For the last 100 years or so, the "virus" has been the scapegoat for diseases—ever since it became glaringly evident that bacteria are of no consequence in the cause of disease, as admitted by Pasteur in his later years. Nevertheless, to this day, physicians cling to the disproven germ theory, although germs in the form of bacteria largely have taken a back seat to the even more elusive "virus."

Chapter 16

THE VIRAL THEORY OF DISEASE CAUSATION

Initially, the word "virus" meant poison, and the word "virulent" meant poisonous. Today, virus means a submicroscopic entity, and virulent generally means contagious. Modern medicine has employed the term virus to mean an ultra-minute form of life that infects cells, and which is blamed for causing more and more of our diseases.

According to the popular portrayal of the virus, it is a form of life that parasitizes all life forms including animal, plant, and saprophytic (fungi and bacteria).

In descriptions of viral disease, viruses are credited with such actions as "injecting themselves," "incubating," "laying in wait," "invading," having an "active stage," "commanding," "re-activating," "disguising themselves," "infecting," "of conducting sieges," and of being "devastating," and "deadly."

Conventional medical theory explains that viruses come from dying cells which they have infected—the virus "injects" itself into the cell and "commands" it to reproduce itself, and this occurs until the cell explodes from the burden. Viruses are then free to seek out other cells to repeat the process, thereby infecting the organism.

Virologists admit, however, that although viruses are distinctive and definitely organic in nature, ***they have no metabolism, cannot be replicated in the laboratory, do not possess any characteristics of living things, and, in fact, have never been observed alive!!***

"Live Viruses" Are Always Dead

The term "live virus" means only those created from living tissue cultures in vitro (within the laboratory) since trillions of them result from "live" tissue. But herein lies the point—**even though some laboratory cultures are kept alive, there is massive cell turnover in the process, and it is from these dying cells that "viruses" are obtained. THEY ARE ALWAYS DEAD AND INACTIVE** because they have no metabolism or life, except being molecules of DNA and protein.

Viruses contain nucleic acid and protein but lack enzymes, and cannot support life on their own since they do not even possess the first prerequisites of life, namely metabolic control mechanisms (and even "lowly" bacteria have these). *Guyton's Medical Textbook* acknowledges that viruses have no reproductive system, no locomotion, no metabolism, and cannot be reproduced as live entities in vitro.

The Mitochondria Connection

Since "viruses" are not alive, they cannot act in any of the ways as ascribed to them by medical authorities except as a functional unit of our *normal* genetic material inside the cell's nucleus or the mitochondrian nucleus within the cell.

Mitochondria are living organisms—just one of many of the varying organelles (little organs) within each cell of our body. Mitochondria are about the size of bacterium, both of which have their own DNA and their own metabolism.

The mitochondria metabolizes glucose into ATP molecules, which is ready made energy usable when called upon by the body. What do these facts have to do with "viruses" as such? EVERYTHING, as you will see in just a moment.

For anyone who has studied cytology (cell structure), the greatest number of life forms within a cell are the mitochondria—the creators of our energy.

Simple single-celled protozoa have up to a half million mitochondria within them. Human cells have less—from a few hundred in blood cells, to 30,000 or more in our larger muscle tissue cells. Since the entire human body contains some 75-100 trillion cells, each containing on the average, thousands of mitochondria, there must be quadrillions or quintillions of them in our system.

When a cell dies, it is replaced by a daughter cell during the process of mitosis, and the spent cell is disintegrated by *lysosomes*—the potent self-destruct, self-digesting, intra-cellular enzymes that break-up cellular components into ultra-minute particles so that the body can readily recycle them or excrete them as waste.

Each day about 300 billion to over 1/2 trillion cells in our body expire (depending on our level of toxicity), each containing an average of 5,000-20,000 mitochondria (some up to 40,000). When cells die they are self-destructed by their own lysosomes but the nuclei and the genomes of mitochondria are better protected than other cellular organelles and protoplasm, and often do not completely decompose.

Genomes and nuclei are microscopic templates of genetic information consisting of DNA or RNA that act as the control center, and the storehouse of the very "blueprints" of the cell. As such, they are to mitochondria and cells what brains are to our body.

Every cell and every mitochondria contains this genetic material which is actually the most protected part of the cell (by virtue of its double-lipid protein sheath) just as our nervous system is the most vital and most protected portion of our physiology (by virtue of our back bone and skull).

Upon cellular death, mitochondria are broken down by lysosomes BUT NOT ALWAYS COMPLETELY, due to their highly protective double-membrane sheath. And here is where this explanation gets interesting.

According to *Guyton's Textbook of Medical Physiology* a virus is said to be a minute bit of genetic material (called a genome) which is literally about a billionth the size of a cell.

The genome is surrounded by a capsid covering that is usually a double/lipid-protein sheath and is actually composed of two unit membranes (almost identical to the cell membrane) which, incidentally, is the very structure of the mitochondrian nucleus.

Photos of "viruses" revealed through electron microscopes show their membranes to be rough and jagged, sometimes only part of one layer and sometimes one layer and a portion of the second, which is consistent with the self-digesting action of lysosomes when their job of breaking down cellular waste is partial and incomplete. As such, this description of a "virus" is virtually identical with the description of the remaining genomes of the cell's *mitochondria* as well.

At one point, viruses were once living matter and some

physiology texts hypothesize that they are the debris of spent cells. Lysosomes that disintegrate the spent cell often fail to break-up these "viruses" surrounded by the double-lipid coat membrane.

It is surprising that researchers fail to recognize these for what they apparently are—spent mitochondrian genetic material, particularly fragments of RNA and DNA.

"Viruses" Are Not Microorganisms

Even though medical authorities mistakenly attribute to this dead cellular debris the powers of life and malevolence, microbiologists acknowledge that viruses are dead bits of DNA in a protein/lipid membrane coat, although failing it realize its source.

Specifically, a genome carries the encoded biochemical information for directing the activities of both the larger cell and the minute mitochondria that resides within it. The genome's encoding helps the living microorganism create energy from glucose, proteins from amino acids, and other basic functions including reproduction, structuring cellular proteins, and for producing operable mitochondria.

As such, *genomes are control mechanisms but NOT microorganisms as the medical establishment would have us believe* since these so-called "viruses" are merely lifeless fragments of mitochondrial genetic debris. Because of this, viruses cannot cause disease unless they accumulate as filth and pollute our cells, tissues, and circulation upon cellular death.

Viruses, then, are dead genomes from disintegrated cells whose cellular membrane is not completely broken down by cellular lysosomes. These genomes apparently come from the nuclei of the cell's vast mitochondrial population which dies along with it, as well as from the nuclei of *megalocytovirus* cells (meaning big virus cell).

Genomes have no characteristics of life whatsoever, and

are merely bits of nucleic acid material normally recycled through phagocytosis or excreted as waste.

Photos of alleged viruses "injecting themselves" into a cell *actually* show the cell literally engulfing the "virus," or proteinaceous debris.

A dent called *invagination* then forms and the organic matter is surrounded by cellular substance which closes off, forming an impromptu stomach, and the "virus" disappears. The stomach then fills with powerful lysosome enzymes which digest the organic material, breaking it down into amino acids and fatty acids for recycling or elimination.

This process is a normal feature of cell physiology called *phagocytosis* (literally cell-eating)—the routine process of cellular ingestion and enzymatic digestion of bacteria, dead tissue debris, and other errant cells.

Viruses are merely inert organic material totally devoid of all life qualities and are *never* seen to act. Photographs purporting to show viruses in action are outright frauds—what is actually shown is an ordinary physiological process of phagocytosis which occurs countless times daily within the body.

Remember, according to medical texts on virology and microbiology, viruses have the following UNLIFELIKE characteristics:

1. Viruses have no metabolism—they cannot process foodstuffs or nutriment an they have no energy formation. *They are only a template, or a pattern of of information as are all genome.*
2. Viruses have no faculties for action of any kind—no nervous system, no sensory apparatus, and no intelligence that may coordinate movement or "bodily invasion" of any kind.
3. Viruses cannot replicate themselves—they supposedly depend wholly upon ***"obligate reproduction"*** —meaning, reproduction by a host organism, SOMETHING TOTALLY UNHEARD OF IN ALL BIOLOGY.

Obligate Reproduction

In the medical rationale to viral disease causation, we are told to believe in *obligate reproduction* , where one organism (the cell) is obligated to reproduce an alien organism (the "virus"). *Nowhere in nature, however, does any living thing reproduce anything other than its own kind.*

Do not forget that the size relationship of a virus to a cell is literally about *one billionth* the size. The viral rationale of disease causation tells us to believe that the virus injects itself into the cell and commands it to reproduce the virus hundreds of thousands of times, upon which the cell explodes.

When the virus "reproduces," its collective mass *STILL equals far less than 1/100th of a percent of the mass of the cell.* That is like saying if you inject yourself with half an ounce of a substance, it will cause so much internal pressure that you will explode!!

This all sounds ridiculous from a biological standpoint since physiology does operate in this manner. "Viruses" by no means cause the cell to explode. Upon normal cellular death, however, the cell does disintegrate, releasing particles of its nucleus of which numerous segments are identified as individual "viruses."

Only living microorganisms are capable of acting and reproducing, which is under direct control of the nucleus, genome, or "brain." A so-called "virus" is a detached part of a once organically functioning entity whose genetic structure has the same relationship that a head has to a body—to ascribe ANY action to viruses is roughly akin to attributing actions to a dead person's decapitated head!

Viruses are not capable of "attacking," "invading," or "infecting" because once the cell dies so does its genetic component. Viruses are particles of dead nuclei that are present in large amounts when body elimination is retarded.

Like all toxins, they harm tissues if not removed promptly through absorption by our cells via normal physiological processes of phagocytosis and pinocytosis (meaning cell-eating and cell-drinking)—*but these processes are completely controlled by cellular intelligence, and NOT by the "virus."* The bottom line is that viruses have no capability of causing anything except further polluting the body.

Viruses Are Toxic Only as Accumulated Wastes

Our blood and tissues may become saturated with these internally generated waste materials, as well as from pollutants ingested from the outside. Intoxication occurs as these overload the body beyond our ability to eject them.

Viruses ***DO*** cause disease in as much as they are toxic waste materials. In this sense, "viruses" do indeed occasion disease BUT NOT AS CONTAGIOUS AGENTS (and this will be addressed at length in the next chapter).

Remember, bacteria, germs, and viruses do not communicate or act in concert and are incapable of conducting joint operations like armies of attackers—they lack the intelligence and resources required to conduct the disease process. Only the body can initiate such a healing crisis since the body is the only unified intelligent entity capable of conducting physiological processes termed "dis-ease."

So-called viruses are toxic in the body as are other debris that clog the body and vitiate it but they do nothing at all in the system for they are completely powerless to act. In spite of this, medical authorities regard viruses as living entities when, in fact, no one has ever observed any quality of life they that ascribe to viruses—***they are always dead!!***

The popular idea that dead organic matter (viruses) can kill off our natural defenses (white blood cells) is nonsense, as these easily guard our blood and fluids from even LIVING yeast and bacterial organisms.

Dead organic material floating in our circulation are readily apprehended, engulfed, digested, and recycled via enzymatic action. Viruses are not alien invaders, but are internally created waste products of cellular decay. Uneliminated, this proteinaceous waste pollutes the circulation and is mislabelled a "virus."

Avoid "Infections" by Living Healthfully

Boyd's Medical Textbook states that most normal persons harbor viruses WITHOUT developing the particular diseases the viruses are supposed to cause, and that enervating influences overcome the body's protective functions, "permitting the viruses to usurp the biological activities within the cell."

More specifically, according to medical theory, for a parasite or virus to be pathogenic it has to meet three criteria:

1. It must be biochemically active—it must have metabolic capacity in order to perform action;
2. It would have to infect or intoxicate *more* of the host's cells than the animal or human organism could spare or regenerate—for instance, you would only suffer from influenza if the virus kills or infects a significant portion of your lung's cells; the polio virus if it affects enough of your nerve cells; or the hepatitis virus if it takes hold of a large portion of your liver cells. (Latent infections are those that involve a small percentage of our cells, like tuberculosis, which most of us have and do not even notice); and
3. The host must be genetically and immunologically permissive. It has to accept the pathogen and cannot be "immune" to it—it has to "let it happen", so to speak.

Medically speaking, infection means invasion by microbial life, *but infection is actually nothing more then toxic materials and decomposed cells concentrated in a particular area by the body for purposes of elimination* .

Infection is commonly defined as "the establishment of a pathogen in a host organism after invasion of an infective agent." The term "pathogen" describes a causative agent of disease (virus or germ) and implies a living organism, although "viruses" are not alive.

Interestingly, toxins are not called "pathogens," yet if anything IS a causative agent of disease, it is ingested toxins which makes US primarily responsible for our own disease suffering.

In fact, humans are always "infected" with bacteria and viruses as they are present in the body at all times—therefore, one cannot say they "invade" the host. Diseases are not infections, rather they are body purification processes and ARE NOT CREATED BY BACTERIA OR "VIRUSES."

Neither "viruses" nor bacteria can cause the illness-/healing crisis. The real culprit is the biologically incorrect lifestyle of the sufferer. When debilitating habits are discontinued there are no further toxic accumulations and the need for the body to generate the healing/disease process will cease to exist. Health is the natural result.

As causes of disease, microbes and genomes ("viruses") are irrelevant because:

1. Healthful living ALWAYS produces health;
2. If acute diseases are suffered, a return to healthful lifestyle practices invariably restores health regardless of their supposed microbial causes;
3. Healthful persons cannot be made sick by exposure to those suffering disease. Children who are reared Hygienically NEVER have the usual "contagious" childhood diseases, although, at times, they too are in constant contact with those who develop measles, chicken pox, mumps, etc.;

4. **Diseases are biological processes specific to a given organism, and cannot be "caught" from someone else, anymore than HEALTH can be "caught" or given to another;** and
5. Healthful living makes one proof against disease. Physicians say the healthy have "high resistance", *which makes germs and viruses irrelevant.* Likewise, they are irrelevant even to those who so enervate themselves that their "resistance is low" since recovery is quickly realized through healthful, drugless measures.

Drugs Are Counterproductive

To kill off bacteria and viruses to enable the body a chance to recover, medics believe, that they must administer drugs. They also believe that medicine assists in healing. Drugs indeed kill off bacteria, but they are just as deadly to all forms of metabolic life, *including human cells* .

The use of drugs and herbal medicines sabotage the body's detoxification efforts by posing an additional threat to the system besides the vile substances it was ejecting via the disease process. Eliminating the newly ingested offending substance now takes precedence over those which caused the healing crisis in the first place.

The medical practice of killing germs with drugs, antibiotics, anti-inflammatory agents, or serums to suppress germ activity is the cause of increasing degeneration of the population and iatrogenic disease.

Acute disease is self-limiting, according to the time and effort required to rid the organism of injurious substances. The work performed by scavenging bacteria during the disease process is both exhausting and unpleasant to the host but is vitally necessary for the preservation of life and health.

After the detoxification process is complete, disease symptoms disappear and the organism again makes its energies amount or normal endeavors. Strength then returns to the extremities. The body, although debilitated from the effort made necessary by its toxic condition, regains its powers and functional vitality and recovers *without* treatment. When the healing crisis is completed, recovery begins.

Almost everyone believes in the "viral theory of disease causation" including all our scientists, both the legitimate ones and those who bask under its invocation.

Most Americans, however, do not actively seek out knowledge independently of what they are told by "authorities," and do not exercise their ability to think and reason enough to know or even suspect that it is impossible for "viruses" to cause anything, other than as pathogenic body waste.

Only when the body is being intoxicated faster than it can detoxify, does toxicosis and its myriad acute and degenerative forms begin to manifest as disease.

Chapter 17

THE ILLUSION OF CONTAGION

Fact or Fiction?

People have been educated to be terrified of bacteria and viruses and to believe implicitly in the idea of *contagion* —that specific malevolently aggressive disease entities pass from one host to another.

Contagion is medically defined as the transmission of disease by contact—an infectious disease is communicable by contact with one suffering from it, or with an object touched by them. The dictionary cites the mechanism as "viruses or other infective agents" or "something that serves as a medium to transmit disease either by direct or indirect means."

Contagion is a medical myth, however, since toxic wastes cannot be passed from one body to the next via normal, contact. The contagious diseases are deceptive, for **no one can give his or her disease to another any more than one**

can give away his or her health. Something *similar* to contagion seems to occur when an extremely toxemic person is exposed to someone similarly ill—thereby triggering a healing crisis.

What's *Really* Going on Here?

Bacteria or germs of such individuals are stimulated into action by those devitalized elements upon which the bacteria thrive.

When transferred to the mucus membranes or tissues of another person EQUALLY toxemic, the bacteria may begin working immediately in the same manner as in the host carrier if adequate decomposition products exist as a food source for bacterial colonies to take hold and thrive. But a soiled environment is a prerequisite to such bacterial action.

The healthy individual with an uncontaminated, relatively pure bloodstream therefore, need not be concerned or apprehensive about "contagious disease."

Once more, only in those persons with a high accumulation of metabolic wastes saturating their tissues and bloodstreams, are their symbiotic bacteria potentially stimulated into action by bacteria transferred from another, equally toxic person.

Only in this sense are diseases "contagious"—the germ precipitates or excites disease in those to whom the germ is transferred, and is a contributing factor in toxic crises in which localized areas of the body are exposed to contamination or "infection." Proper soil (food) is thereby provided and bacteria proliferate exponentially.

But malevolent bacteria, germs, and/or "viruses" are not the primary cause of disease, rather a polluted body is.

We usually cannot transfer our toxic load to someone else unless it is drawn out of us (as in donating blood) and then injected into another person (as in transfusion). This represents medically induced contagion or iatrogenic disease, rather than those occurring within the realm of natural biological life processes. Serums or drugs help add to the general toxic load, and instability results in serious chronic illness later in life.

This is the true explanation of "contagion". ***The germ triggers, precipitates or excites the disease process in those who are toxemic.*** **But in those who are not, contagion is not valid and does not exist so long as the body is pure—for it is the soil in the system that prepares the body for "contagions" by our failure to keep our body fluids and tissues clean and non-polluted.**

The *Actual* "Contagious" Factors and Influences

In reality, there is no such thing as "contagion," for the only disease producing agents are biologically unhealthful habits such as indulgence in alcohol, coffee, cigarettes, drugs, junk foods, refined foods, too little rest and sleep, lack of exercise and sunshine, etc.

Bacteria, germs, and viruses are incapable of causing disease, **as these only result from an unsanitary condition within the body and are present in disease NOT AS CAUSATIVE AGENTS but as the result of unhygienic conditions.**

It is the biologically incorrect lifestyle practices which cause diseases that are rampant throughout the population. **It is NOT any "bug that is going around", it is what we do to our own body that violates its systemic needs.**

The great bubonic plagues of the past, and the AIDS epidemic of today are NOT due to contagion. Epidemics appear to exist because the true contagions are the similar biologically poor lifestyle habits shared by virtually all. As a population, people pretty much consume the same types of junk food; people generally indulge in very similar health-compromising practices (lack of rest, inadequate exercise, constantly using drugs and stimulants, etc.); people are subjected to the same seasonal changes; and live pretty much in the same type of housing.

Similar afflictions run rampant when those suffering them indulge in similar poor lifestyle routines. Similar bad habits, in other words, beget similar bad results.

Look at it this way—if 100 people take an emetic and those 100 people vomit, it might be concluded that vomiting is very contagious. All this actually proves, however, is that "similar organisms subjected to similar influences react similarly." **The *only* contagions are the same poor habits that manifest in basically the same diseases.**

In nature, for instance, we were not gluttons—we did not eat contrary to our biological adaptations. Instead we ate instinctively, did not intoxicate our systems, nor did we suffer disease just as animals in nature do not get sick when in their natural environment, unspoiled by man.

Like causes beget like effects—it is no wonder that many suffer the same diseases modified of course, by the weaknesses of each individual. This is why, within the context of a given family or community, people who share the same poor lifestyle habits also suffer similar diseases. **It is not germ or viral contagion, but pathogenic conditions that create so-called epidemics or plagues.**

Diseases "get around" because the pathological practices that beget illness are themselves widespread. The only true contagions are the widespread modes of improper sanitation, and the destructive lifestyle routines that are now, and have been previously common-place—specifically in this country, the constant stress factors; the constant drugging; and the constant poison habits that we subject ourselves to.

Meat eating is widespread. Refined sugar use is widespread. Coffee drinking is widespread. Lack of adequate rest and sleep, and breathing polluted air is widespread, and so on. In this light, so-called "contagion" is caused by the insalubrious society in which we live.

Alcohol, cigarettes, drugs, medicines, biologically improper foods, lack of pure water, fresh air, etc., all produce the diseases we suffer from. Live healthfully and there are no contagious diseases. It is as simple as adhering to our natural mandate.

But Why Isn't Everyone Sick?

As practiced wholesale by the population at large, unhealthful lifestyles produce generally the same vulnerable and susceptible conditions in great numbers of people who, through intimate contact, can conceivably trigger disease symptoms in each other.

BUT DON'T BE FOOLED. What about the thousands who develop cold and flu symptoms who have NOT been in contact with someone suffering similarly? And what about the thousands **WHO ARE** in intimate contact with those who are ill, **BUT DO NOT** get sick?

Remember, disease is a self-initiated cleansing process—an extraordinary eliminative effort created by the body when it can no longer tolerate a toxemic internal condition.

Constructive diseases are biological processes of detoxification and repair, and only acute or constructive diseases are said to be "contagious." Expose a truly healthy person to all the diseases of humanity AND THEY WILL NOT BE AFFECTED. Actually, neither will an unhealthy person be affected since all acute diseases are body initiated and conducted conditions.

Why is it that some who are exposed to so-called "contagious disease" are subsequently laid low themselves, while others similarly exposed are not? The answer lies in the fact that those who maintain an internal state of cleanliness via biologically correct habits of eating and living do not require the disease process—it cannot develop unless the toxic conditions preexist and favor its manifestation.

"Susceptibility"

The concept of "contagion" is closely related to the equally erroneous notion of "susceptibility"—for a contagion is supposedly "contagious" only if the individual is "susceptible." This medical rationale is really an admission that germs do not cause disease. If they did, everyone exposed would become sick with the same disease.

Actually, a "susceptible" person is one with a high degree of body toxicity, along with the sufficient vitality to conduct the disease/purification process. The individual may become ill whether exposed to a "contagion" or not *at any given time* .

When truly healthy individuals maintain their health *while in the midst of "communicable or epidemic diseases,"* then it must be self-evident that the theory of contagion is incorrect.

Keep in mind, different diseases are varying symptom complexes that arise out of reduced nerve energy and increased toxicity. Lifestyle patterns that waste nerve energy result in inhibition of secretion and excretion, which in turn, causes consequent self-poisoning.

The part of the body most laden with toxins is the first to exhibit disease symptoms, but the overall effect is systemic as all the organs and glands of the system suffer impairment to some degree.

We must realize, however, that sickness is not an enemy. Discomforts and acute symptoms are the body's warning signals during detoxification that we are somehow living in such a way that is contrary to our natural mandate.

So long as we heed these signals in a timely manner by resting and fasting rather than waiting for a full-fledged healing crisis, the body will usually require a much briefer and relatively mild cleansing period. So long as we keep the system pure in this manner, we need not fear "contagion" or "epidemics."

Colds, flu, leprosy, measles, chicken pox, AIDS, etc., are said to be contagious while meningitis, polio-myelitis, asthma, psoriasis, cancer, and a long list of other diseases have been removed from the contagious list.

Ignorance regarding the true nature of disease, however, is about the only true contagion there is. Remember, disease is a body initiated and conducted process, and is not caused by germs that attack those who are "susceptible."

Take colds for instance. How is it that infants have about eight colds per year while the parents only a few? How is it that those persons isolated at observation posts in the North and South Poles "catch" colds during their stay? How is it that between 1965-67 the National Institute of Health's cold laboratories in Bethesda, Maryland conducted experiments that showed everything but contagion?

Volunteers were swabbed daily with supposed cold "viruses" taken directly from those suffering colds, and none became ill. *More in the control group developed colds.* In the meantime, shortly following traditional Thanksgiving feasts, the number of colds in both groups increased dramatically as would be expected when excessively rich food and drink is consumed during holiday festivities.

Venereal disease is also supposed to be contagious—but the so-called contagious factors (bacteria) are present BECAUSE of the disease and ARE NOT THE CAUSE of the condition (and 20% or so of those suffering V.D. have neither gonococcus or spirochetes which are said to cause it).

The U.S. Navy conducted experiments which showed that so-called "infected persons" could not infect those termed healthy. In Japan, "infected" prostitutes had been with dozens of G.I.s, none of whom contracted the disease. Similarly, many individuals *have* "infections" in the genital area who have not been in contact with anyone (as seen in cases involving young children). The concept of contagion is medically unproven despite appearances to the contrary.

And How About Our True "Epidemics?"

Furthermore, the MOST prevalent diseases around ARE NOT EVEN CONTAGIOUS. Over 90% of all Americans have plaque in their arteries, yet this is not considered contagious. (But AIDS which IS declared to be an epidemic affects only 1/10,000th the number of people)!! Is obesity considered contagious? It effects one of every three people. How about constipation—it affects about 90% of our population.

And is bad eyesight which affects two of every three persons contagious? The same can be said for bad teeth, high blood pressure, headaches, lower back problems, etc., as these diseases are extremely widespread. More than half of all Americans have cardiovascular problems, but are they contagious? The most feared of all diseases is cancer. Is it contagious? Arthritis affects more people than herpes. Is it contagious? And how about asthma and acne?

The Bottom Line

So-called "contagious diseases" like AIDS, venereal disease, and athlete's foot are no more contagious than any other disease—but it does serve certain commercial interests *to make people believe* that they are.

Take herpes, for example. While herpes of the lip area (which is NOT represented as being contagious) is no different than herpes of the genital area except for location there is much medical and religious mileage—the kind that translates into money and power—gained from social and psychological persecution of those whose body's have elected to eliminate extraordinary toxic loads through the genital area.

Basically, acceptance of the theory of contagion is contingent upon acceptance of the germ theory of disease—that specific bacteria or "viruses" *produce* specific disease symptoms. This theory has been repeatedly demonstrated as incorrect in the scientific field, and was even admitted by Pasteur as being incorrect.

Nevertheless, the germ theory and the theory of contagion are perpetuated by our modern medical system whose prestige, profits, and power are largely based on belief in this erroneous theory.

The belief in contagion is difficult to overcome since almost everyone's mind has been similarly "infected" by exploitive "health care" industries that have a vested interest in disease and suffering and in perpetuating such erroneous beliefs.

Basically, the populace believes what the medical establishment wants it to. The theory of contagion maintains the demand for their drug, medical, and hospital practices.

If you live healthfully you will likely never suffer disease, just as Hygienic children never suffer the "usual childhood diseases." **Diseases are caused only by unhealthful lifestyle practices.**

Do not forget, ***only*** the drug, hospital, and medical industries teach that health is recovered by administering poisonous drugs. THIS perhaps is one of the most prominent seeds of "contagious" disease.

The bottom line is that IF germs play any role in the causation of disease, it is never a primary one but is always secondary to those causes that lower our resistance or impair health.

Good health is the maximum insurance against all disease in all cases. The primary cause of illness is the sum of those antecedent factors responsible for the initial impairment of health—this is why we proclaim "health through healthful living."

SECTION VI

FOR THOSE SINCERELY SEEKING HEALTH

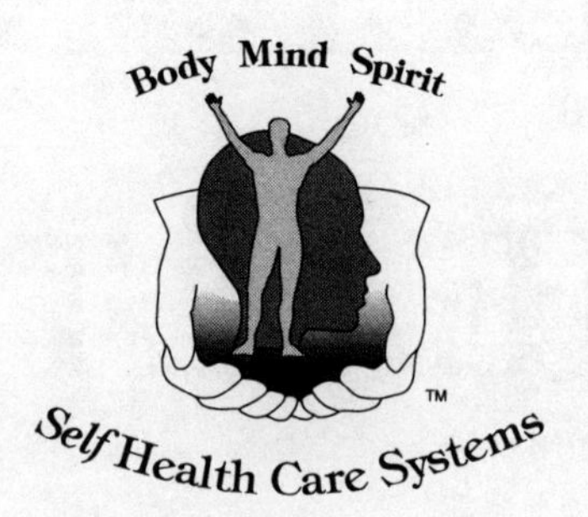
Body Mind Spirit
TM
Self Health Care Systems

Chapter 18

TO GENERATE HEALTH, *ACTION* IS REQUIRED TO CREATE IT— AND WHY WE MUST

It is extremely important that everyone who desires health, understands how it is built and maintained. Each of us must be allowed the freedom of choice in health care and must be allowed the opportunity to construct a rational model of health that is consistent with how the biological realm operates.

With ***this*** information of the nature of our **Self**-healing body, we now have this opportunity. Each of us now has a choice to make, which will largely determine the quality of our life.

Never static, the human body is always in a dynamic state of flux—it either develops greater health, or atrophies towards disease. Change is constant until death ends the cohesion of our body. We build and maintain health only by continually refining our habits and by living in accord with our essential nature.

Natural Hygiene returns to the individual CONTROL over one's health and quality of life, and places one largely in control of his or her own destiny. Lifestyle that is in accord with our biological disposition is the foundation of health, that which is contrary to our nature provides the basis of disease.

HEALTH IS NOT A GIFT OF GOD, AND ILLNESS IS NOT A STROKE OF BAD LUCK—for these are creations of our own making, based on conditions we largely choose and build by ourselves.

Those who sincerely desire superb health must do more than wish for it—they must make a lifetime commitment to their own well-being.

Hygienic Health Care has created entirely new possibilities in the field of health—regarding our ability to remove and prevent disease, to preserve youthfulness, and to significantly lengthen not only life itself, but, more importantly, the QUALITY OF LIFE.

By removing most disease manifestations, through preventing some 95% of their occurrences, a QUALITY life span of 100-150 years is the probable result—accompanied by a painless death, usually during sleep, as seen in nature throughout the animal kingdom.

Animal species in their natural habitat live around seven times their age of maturity. For humans who live in harmony with their biological mandate, this comes to 100-150 quality years of life.

No longer are we justified in dividing diseases into curable and non-curable types, nor in speaking of the inevitable senility and degenerative conditions ordinarily seen in our elderly.

The continuing full and complete implementation of the Hygienic Health Care System within hundreds of thousands of individuals over its history, in addition to extensive observations and studies in the fields of physiology, biology, chemistry, anthropology, paleontology, zoology, and anthropogenesis, provides a sound scientific basis for these possibilities.

It is the role of Hygienic Self-Health Care to teach people how to prevent disease, not merely how to care for themselves when ill.

Hygiene is well aware of the revolutionary change in health care, and in society as well, that the implementation of these methods will bring about—but with the growing incidence of deadly chronic diseases such as AIDS, the health of our entire race may depend upon their acceptance.

A growing number of Americans are becoming disillusioned with conventional medicine and are seeking health guidance elsewhere. The dismal lack of success of life-threatening "cures," and the prospect of having an entire life's savings wiped out during the maltreatment of disease, is sobering.

The time is ripe for a revolutionary change in health care—not merely reform or compromise, but for true SELF-HEALTH CARE to replace our prevailing "disease-care" system.

Just as the late Dr. Herbert M. Shelton alluded to, economy alone should cause the public to adopt Hygienic Health Care, for its adoption by our population would save millions if not billions of dollars yearly in physician bills, prescription bills, hospital bills insurance costs, and time missed from work. The enormous tax burden that our citizens bear to maintain public health organizations would be lifted—and this enormous tax saving is small, compared to the suffering that its adoption would circumvent.

And In Closing.........

For those individuals ready to make the transition to biologically correct living, you are about to make the greatest decision in your life. **Your challenge is this: PERSEVERE.**

Do not become distressed by symptoms of detoxification that may manifest. Instead, learn about your body and how it purifies itself—by reading books and listening to educational tapes, all available through the numerous Natural Hygiene organizations in the United States and around the world (see appendix A for listings). Soon enough, symptoms of healing subside, energy increases, and lasting health is realized as long as healthful living is implemented.

The body is the greatest health-generating machine ever constructed. When we learn to work WITH it by answering its simple needs, it provides a vehicle for fulfillment beyond our fondest dreams.

And *our* reward as Hygienic practitioners, is to impart what has been learned over the decades. This is an ongoing effort, to understand and continuously apply the most challenging of all studies—the science and art of healthful living.

APPENDICES

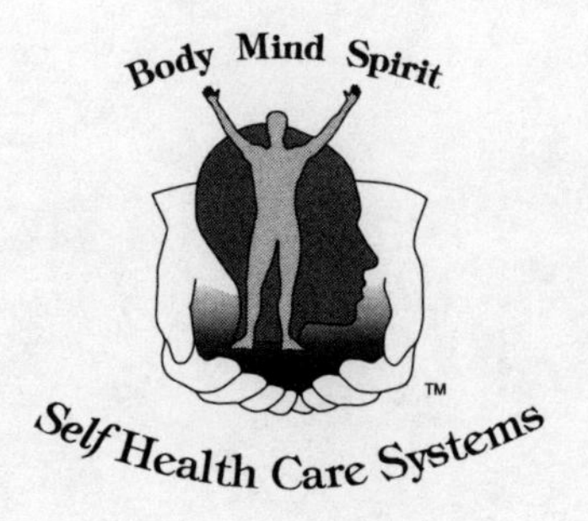
Body Mind Spirit
TM
Self Health Care Systems

Appendix A

ORGANIZATIONS OF NATURAL HYGIENE

American Natural Hygiene Society
P.O. Box 30630, Tampa, FL 33630

Canadian Natural Hygiene Society
Joe Aaron, P.O. Box 235, Station T
Toronto, Canada M6B 4A1

British Natural Hygiene Society
Dr. Keki Sidhwa, Shalimar Retreat,
3 Harold Grove, Frinton-on-the-Sea, Essex,
England, United Kingdom

Australian Natural Hygiene Society
Cobah Road—Arcadia, N.S.W. 2159 AUSTRALIA

Natural Hygiene Inc.
Jo Willard, P.O. Box 2132, Huntington, CT 06484

Health Excellence Systems
(formerly Life Science Institute)
T.C. Fry, 1108 Regal Row, Manchaca, Texas 78652

Bionomics Health Research Institute
Drs. Elizabeth and Robert McCarter,
P.O. Box 36107, Tucson, AZ 85470

GetWell StayWell America
Victoria Bidwell, 1776 The Hygiene Joy Way,
Mount Vernon, WA 98273

Hygienic Community Network
P.O. Box 7972, Santa Cruz, California 95060

Fit For Life
2210 Wilshire Blvd., Suite 118, Santa Monica, CA
90403

Appendix B

THE HISTORY OF NATURAL HYGIENE

Similar to today, back in the early 1800s at the dawn of Natural Hygiene, *results* in matters of public health care were missing—and *also* led to health reform in that early era of our country's history.

The following is a brief description of the general life-style habits of the early 1800's:

- Fresh air, cold air, night air and drafts are feared by the public;
- Houses are unventilated and stale air is trapped in-doors. Closed windows prevent sunlight from entering, and sanitation is generally neglected;
- Nearly all men chew tobacco—and alcohol, coffee, and tea are the adult beverages of choice. Meat, bread, grains, and lard pies are the favored diet while uncooked fruits and vegetables are neglected;

- Life expectancy is about 60 years;
- Common illnesses include cholera, malaria, typhoid, dysentery, pneumonia, TB, typhus, yellow fever, among numerous others; and
- Medical doctors practice indiscriminate bleeding and bloodsucking with leeches of one to two pints of blood for almost all illnesses. Physicians also regularly burn, blister, and cauterize the site where disease disease is thought to harbor within the body. People fear these methods, and desire a health care system that is neither frightening, painful, nor deadly.

Over 175 years ago, as mentioned in chapter four, Dr. Jennings, Trall, Graham, and other disenchanted physicians began publicly challenging the medical approach to health care. These early Natural Hygienists, instead, advocated fresh air and sunshine, good diet, and the avoidance of "social poisons" including tobacco, alcohol, and coffee in the treatment of disease.

In its modern phase, Natural Hygiene is the product of the accumulated knowledge acquired by pioneering Hygienic practitioners. The system was never "discovered," as such, but simply developed year by year, decade by decade through continued experience and observation in healing the sick.

The knowledge gained from this experience formed the basis of a new array of publications which have been released intermittently up to the present day. Included among these are the following publications (listed by author)—and though this listing represents only a fraction of those published, the following publications have exerted the greatest influence in developing the Hygienic System to its present position:

- *Medical Reform, Philosophy of Human Life and Tree of Life or Human Degeneracy, Its Nature and Remedy as Based on the Elevating Principles of Orthopathy* by Isaac Jennings, M.D.;

- *The Hygienic System; Hydropathic Encyclopedia; The Hygienic Handbook; Popular Physiology; Scientific Basis of Vegetarianism* (and numerous others) by Russell Thacker Trall, M.D.;
- *Health From Diet and Exercise; Nature's Own Book;* and *Lectures on the Science of Human Life* by Sylvester Graham;
- *How to Treat the Sick Without Drugs; Hygienic Medication or Science Versus Speculation;* and *Nature's Method of Curing the Sick* by James C. Jackson, M.D.
- *The Nutritive Cure; Hygienic Hydropathy; Exact Science of Health; Life's Great Law; Philosophy of Health Reform; A Defense of Hygienic Treatment; How Sick People Are Cured;* and *Drug Medicines as Causes of Disease* by Robert Walter, M.D.;
- *The Bible of Nature; Mind and Body; Physical Education and Fasting;* and *Hydrotherapy and Exercise* by Felix L. Oswald;
- *Paralysis and Other Afflictions of the Nerves;* and *An Exposition of the Swedish Movement Cure* by George H. Taylor;
- *Life and Health or the Laws and Means of Physical Culture* by William A. Alcott, M.D.
- *Drugless Medicine* by Susanna W. Dodds, M.D.;
- *The Natural Cure* by Charles E. Page;
- *How Nature Cures and Natural Cure of Consumption* by Emmet Densmore;
- *The No-Breakfast Plan; Fasting Cure;* and *The True Science of Living* by Edward Hooker Dewey, M.D.;
- *The Genesis and Control of Disease* by George S. Weger, M.D.;
- *Criticisms of the Practice of Medicine; Impaired Health;* and *Toxemia Explained* by John H. Tilden, M.D.; and

- *The Hygienic System* (seven volumes) by Dr. Herbert M. Shelton

Since the time of Jennings, Trall, and Graham, Natural Hygiene has been the victim of attacks—many by commercial enterprises who see a danger to their vested interests.

Exponents of Hygiene, to this day, are labeled faddists, cultists and quacks, some have been mobbed while lecturing, and many have been heavily fined and even imprisoned for employing Hygienic methods—while being accused of either practicing medicine without a license, or of treating disease other than via established medical means.

Medical and pharmaceutical interests have been particularly active in fighting Hygienic Self-Health Care and have frequently sought to prevent Hygienic practitioners from practicing.

As in other commercial enterprises, medical science sees in Natural Hygiene a threat to its financial interests which, no doubt, is partly responsible for its antagonistic attitude. In the meantime, however, medical science has never made any official investigation to determine the results of Natural Hygiene.

Had Hygienic Health Care been deemed commercially profitable, it might have been absorbed into medical practice. But since people get well and *end* their need for the physician and his drugs, Hygiene is not only non-profitable but is downright unhealthy for the bottom line and bad for business.

Nevertheless, the best-selling health and diet book in history *Fit For Life* (well over eleven million copies sold) popularized Natural Hygiene worldwide in the mid-1980s.

The book is now available in 32 countries and has been translated into 24 languages. Since 1985, when the book was initially published, it has sold over 200,000 copies by word of mouth alone without any additional advertising or publicity.

Currently, *Fit For Life* is experiencing phenomenal success in Europe, especially in Germany where it has recently sold well over one million copies in a country whose population is but a fraction of that in the U.S. This phenomenal success rests on the fact that the program works and is recommended by those who try it.

A brief history of this phenomenon, and of Natural Hygiene itself is outlined below:

1822—Dr. Isaac Jennings having practiced medicine for 20 years and having become thoroughly discouraged with the results, goes undercover and administers placebos of bread pills, starch powders, and colored water tonics to patients, while instructing them in healthful living.

1822-1832—Dr. Jennings and physiologist-minister Sylvester Graham start a healing system called "Orthopathy," and the health reform movement in this country begins. During the following few decades, a group of health-conscious doctors and citizens boldly claim that Nature knows better than the most learned physicians, regarding what is needed to generate and maintain health.

The people of this country are fed-up with the failures and contradictions of current medical practice and theory. For this reason, the truths proclaimed by Jennings and Graham find immediate and widespread acceptance. Before long, Dr. Jenning's fame increases, as his healing record is truly remarkable.

After becoming fully convinced of the correctness of his "Let-Alone Plan," "Do-Nothing Cure," and the "No-Medicine Plan," Jennings announces his discovery to the world—but he is misunderstood, and his message is ill-received. His pioneering impact, however, is felt, and to this day Jennings is credited with being "The Father of Natural Hygiene."

1830-1832—The charismatic minister and physiologist Sylvester Graham, while delivering a seemingly innocent lecture at a Pennsylvania Temperance Society meeting, declares war on prevailing medical practices and earns the title "Father of the Philosophy of Physiology."

For several years Graham lectures nationwide on the relationship of physiology to Hygiene and gains a large following, especially among the common working people. In just a few years, he publishes *"The Graham Journal of Health and Longevity;"* establishes the Library of the American Physiologic Society; opens the nation's first health food stores, health book stores, and health food restaurants; and founds numerous "Grahamit" health retreats and boarding houses.

1833—Dr. Russell Thacker Trall emerges as a great mastermind of Hygienic "Hygieo-Therapy," which combines the use of all Hygienic agents into one holistic system. A brilliant thinker and articulate debater, Dr. Trall publicly challenges the medical establishment on their theory and practice and always comes out the victor.

1844—Dr. Joel Shew introduces the European system of "Hydrotherapy" to the United States, a curing treatment which uses little or no drugs while employing water as the main therapeutic agent. Hydropathists adopt the Hygieo-Therapy dietary and exercise plan, as well as its emphasis on fresh air and sunlight. American physicians who had lost faith in drugging but lacked belief in Hygiene adopt Hydrotherapy wholesale as both become intertwined and indistinguishable for several years.

1830-1860— Scores of Hygienic homes, Schools and Sanitariums open throughout the country. Dr. Harriet Austin and James Jackson found the largest Natural Hygiene institution in the world, "Our Home on the Hillside" boasting 250 beds. Seventy-five hydrotherapy (water-cure) institutions are founded. During this time, over 80 "health papers" effectively reach the masses which coincide with an improvement in the hygienic habits of Americans.

1852—Natural Hygiene is so enthusiastically received and popularized that its practitioners outnumber those of allopathic, homeopathic, chiropractic, and eclectic medicine.

1853—Dr. Russell Trall founds the New York College of Hygieo-Therapy to educate competent health practitioners. This inaugurates a new era in medical science—in theory, philosophy and practice—that is in variance with prevailing allopathic doctrines of the time.

1861—Trall, who had once been a practicing Hydropathist, announces a formal declaration separating Hydrotherapy from Hygieo-Therapeutics (Natural Hygiene) by stating "water possesses no power whatsoever to cure any disease. Nature is the remedial principle."

1862—Trall delivers a landmark lecture at the Smithsonian Institute in Washington D.C. before the most distinguished medical minds in this country entitled "The True Healing Art, or Hygiene vs. Medication." The lecture is widely published and circulated among the populace, and the health reform movement in this country reaches its height. Ironically, in 1861, with the onset of the Civil War, national attention focuses on survival—and health reform ends.

1861-1865—The Civil War causes Hygienic institutions everywhere to close. The health reform movement is halted as the war impoverishes the nation. Schools and sanitariums are wrecked and the common citizen can no longer afford Hygienic educational literature.

1864—French chemist Louis Pasteur fathers "The Science of Bacteriology" and "The Germ Theory of Disease" by demonstrating the existence of microorganisms. It is concluded that "germs" cause pathogenic change in living cultures within laboratory experiments.

With Pasteur, a new era in modern medicine is inaugurated, including sterilization, pasteurization, vaccination, and fear of raw foods. The prevailing "germ era" helps usher in the decline of 19th century health reform. Not only did people develop germ-phobia, but they also found complacency in blaming their ill-health on malevolent invading bacteria, rather than taking responsibility for their own poor lifestyle choices.

1881—Clara Barton, student of Hygiene and friends of Drs. Harriet Austin and James Jackson, founds the American Red Cross and becomes its first president.

1900-1940—Dr. J. H. Tilden, after thoroughly reading 19th century Hygienic literature, becomes convinced that disease need not be experienced. Tilden conducts a private practice to teach patients how to eliminate body toxicity; he lectures widely; writes 25 books; and widely circulates a monthly magazine both in this country and abroad.

1909-1910—The infamous *Flexner Report* ends health-care reform in this country, as alternative schools of healing are shutdown nationwide under the influence of the Rockefeller and Carnegie Foundations (see chapter #1 for details).

1924-1940—Tilden opens and operates a Hygienic school and sanitarium in Denver, Colorado. In 1926, he publishes the famous book *"Toxemia Explained"*, which identifies the primary cause of all disease as toxemia (a state of internal pollution) brought on by enervating, unhealthful living. In the meantime, medical authorities strongly oppose and condemn Tilden.

1920—Dr. Herbert M. Shelton writes the first of 40 books in his effort to revive Natural Hygiene. Over the next 50 years, many of Dr. Shelton's books are translated into eight languages.

1928-1981—Dr. Shelton's Health School operates in San Antonio, Texas and includes a clinic, laboratory, and educational program. People receive care, and well over 40,000 fasts are professionally supervised, while, according to Shelton, "the sick get well, the well get better, and all gain the priceless knowledge needed to stay well." Throughout his career, Shelton is considered a threat to medicine. He is repeatedly threatened and even jailed over 30 times.

1948—The American Natural Hygiene Society is founded. Several chiropractors and laymen elect Shelton as its first president. Annual conventions are held, and 30 chapters worldwide are established—some of which are active today. Current membership in the U.S., however, is below 10,000.

1939-1980—Shelton publishes the monthly magazine *Hygienic Review* popularizing and reviving Natural Hygiene worldwide for 20th century thinkers. From 1934-1941, Shelton also wrote and published the seven-volume series entitled *The Hygienic System,* which becomes the basis for Hygienic study in this century.

1970—At age 44, Terrance C. Fry reads Shelton's book "Superior Nutrition" and becomes a hygienist overnight. Within a few years, he writes and self-publishes several easy-to-read booklets and books popularizing Natural Hygiene, that are in contrast to Shelton's formidable textbooks and manuals of sophisticated vocabulary. Fry's books serve to prime inspired readers for some of Shelton's more complex reading.

1982—T.C. Fry founds Life Science Institute and publishes *Healthful Living* magazine with a circulation of 30,000. Fry also develops a Natural Hygiene teacher-training course, a 2200 page, 111-lesson home study curriculum that enrolls well over 2,000 students worldwide. Life Science Institute also produces audio and video cassettes on Natural Hygiene and offers retreats and seminars to students and to the general public.

1983—Dr. Shelton loses his Health School after being sued for malpractice. In 1985, Shelton dies.

1986-1988—Harvey and Marilyn Diamond, after years of study with Life Science Institute and counseling and teaching, write ***Fit For Life***—the best-selling health and diet book in history. A second book ***Living Health*** follows. Warners Brothers publishes and provides extensive national coverage through media and conferences, which popularizes Natural Hygiene for millions of Americans.

1990s—Many Hygienic organizations and practitioners continue operating educational programs, retreats, sanitariums, and private practices, although relatively few are directed by those with "recognized" credentials.

Appendix C

PRACTITIONERS OF NATURAL HYGIENE

The first listing is the membership of the **International Association of Professional Natural Hygienists.** All members are primary care doctors licensed and/or legally practicing in their state, country or territory.

Charisse Basquin, D.C.
2900 St. Paul Dr. #219
Santa Rosa, CA 95405
(907) 456-6213

Gerald Benesh D.C.
2050 Rockhoff Rd.,
Escondido, CA 92026
(619) 747-4193

John Brosious B.S., D.C.
18209 Gulf Blvd.,
Redington Shores, FL 33708
(813) 392-8326

Trevor Salloum N.D.
557 Bernard Ave.
Kelowna B.C., CANADA
(604) 763-5445

D.J. Scott D.C.
P.O. Box 361095
Strongsville, OH 44136
(216) 671-5023

Keki R. Sidwa N.D.
Shalimar—Harold Grove
Frinton-on-the-Sea
ENGLAND CO139BD
(phone) 011-44-25-567-2823

Nejla Burton, D.O.
Alec Burton M.Sc., D.O.,
Arcadia Health Centre
Cobah Road—Arcadia, N.S.W.
2159 AUSTRALIA
(phone) Sydney 653-1115

Ralph C. Cinque D.C.
Hygeia Health Retreat
439 East Main
Yorktown, Texas 78164
(512) 564-3670

Peter Coumentakis N.D.
Theodora Coumentakis M.D.
Palaion Polemiston 30, Glyfada,
Attici GREECE
962-2387

Ronald G. Cridland M.D.
Health Promotion Clinic
9955 Younge St. Ste #102,
Richmond Hill,Ontario,
CANADA L4C 9M6

William Esser N.D., D.C.
Esser's Health Ranch
P.O. Box 6229,
Lake Worth, FL 33466
(407) 965-4360

Douglas F. Evans D.O.
P.O. Box 78, Culburra Beach,
New South Wales 2540
AUSTRALIA
(phone) 044-472-081

Stanley S. Bass D.C.,
3119 Coney Islands Ave.
Brooklyn, NY 11235
(718) 648-1500

Pierre Cloutier D.C.
10 Rue Bell, Chateauguay
Quebec, CANADA J6J 3L8
(514) 691-1102

Jacque Dezavelle D.C.
1118 Second St.
Encinitas, CA 92024
(619) 436-5151

Greg Fitzgerald D.O.,
1/31-33 Geralle St.
Cronulla, Sydney 2230
AUSTRALIA
(phone) 523-2108

Joel Fuhrman M.D.
450 Amwell Rd.
Belle Mead, NJ 08502
(908) 359-1775

Doug Graham D.C.
Club Hygiene
105 Bruce Court
Marathon, FL 33050
(305) 743-3168

Thomas K. Hand
3676 Richmond Ave.
Staten Island, NY 10312
(718) 984-5869

David Engle D.C.
Alan Goldhammer D.C.
Alec Isabeau D.C.
Jennifer Marano D.C.
Center for Chiropractic and Conservative Therapy
4310 Lichau Rd.,
Penngrove, CA 94951
(707) 792-2325

Philip Martin D.C.
15 Ridge Hill Dr., Toronto,
Ontario, CANADA M6C 2J2
(416) 482-2340

Frank Sabatino D.C., Ph.D
Regency Health Resort and Spa
2000 S. Ocean Dr.,
Hallendale, FL 33009
(305) 454-4004

Guy Harris D.O.
4-12-4 Minami
Nagaski, Toshima-ku
Tokyo 171, JAPAN

Steve Nelson D.C.
7340 Ulmerton Rd.
Largo, FL 33541
(813) 535-7754

Thomas Nocun M.D.
Hutnicza 18/44
20-218 Lublin
POLAND

Dan Keret M.D.
7 Haparsa St.
Zahala, 69085
ISRAEL

Additional doctors across the country who incorporate Natural Hygiene into their practice include the following:

Norman Allard D.C.
323 N. Wisconsin St.
Gunnison, CO 81230
(303) 641-4044

Paul W. Carlin II D.C.
711 Bay Area Blvd.
Webster, TX 77598
(713) 332-1111

Christopher Deatherage D.C.
Star Route, Box 87A
Chamis, MO 65024
(314) 943-2282

David L. Reichel D.C.
330 West Main
Perham, MN 56573
(218) 346-2330

Dr. Joel Robbins
Health and Wellness
6218 South Lewis, Ste 103
Tulsa, OK. 74136
(918) 742-2194

Philip C. Royal D.C.
2607 De La Vina St.
Santa Barbara, CA 93105
(805) 569-1702

Stephen Forest D.C.
430 Monteray Ave #2
Los Gatos, CA 95030
(408) 358-2188

Robert Gross D.C. Ph.D
Pawling Health Manor
P.O. Box 401
Hyde Park, NY 12538
(914) 889-4141

Alan Immerman D.C.
Immerman Chiropractic
5743 E. Thomas Rd. Suite #2
Scottsdale, AZ 85251
(602) 946-1597

Paul Levy D.C.
6144 W. Roosevelt Rd.,
Oak Park, IL 60304
(213) 865-2533

Anthony J. Penepent M.D.
2-12 W. Park Ave.
P.O. Box 886
Long Beach, NY 11561
(718) 834-2330

Leslie H. Salov M.D.
Vision and Health Center
Rte. 4, Box 186
Whitewater, WI 53190
(414) 473-7361

Dr. Henry Stephenson
The Euphorium
563-D Street SW
Corvallis, OR 97333
(503) 755-7154

Andrew Vitko D.C.
17023 Loraine Ave.
Cleveland, OH 44111
(216) 671-5023

Dr. Weiss D.C.
409 E. Front Street
Bloomington, IL 61701
(309) 452-3921

John McDougall M.D.
St. Helena Hospital Center
Deer Park, CA 94576
(800) 862-7575

The following retreats also offer Natural Hygiene Health-Care (in addition to those already listed) around the United States:

Mary Kelly
Ron Schade
GetWell/StayWell
America's Last Resort
1001 North Browne Ave.
Brownsville, TX 78521
(512) 831-5218

Bernice Davison
The Health Oasis
Rte. #2, Box 10
Tilly, AR 72679
(501) 496-2364

John Peet
God's Own Sanctuary of Health
H.C.R. 642
Payton, AZ 85521
(602) 474-2220

Mort Pine
Regency Health Resort and Spa
2000 South Ocean Dr.
Hallandale, FL 33009
(918) 742-2194

Dr. Tosca Vetrano
Revitalization &
Rejuvenation Retreat
P.O. Box 212
Barksdale, TX 78828
(210) 234-3499

Rhoda Mozorosky
The Umpqua House of Oregon
7338 Oak Hill Rd.
Roseburg, OR 97470
(503) 459-4700

The Born Again Body Hideaway
P.O. Box 660
Covelo, CA 95528
(707) 983-8323

Jean Schnake
The Russell House
116 Truman Ave.
Key West, FL 33040
(305) 294-8787

David Cheatam
Shangri-La
P.O. Box 2328
Bonita Springs, FL 33959
(813) 992-3811

Helen LaMar
Unlimited Vision
556 Sunlit Lane
Santa Cruz, CA 95060
(408) 426-8546

Helena Henn
Helena's Health Haven
1105 Patterson Lane
Pacific Grove, CA 93950
(408) 373-1119

Oleta Thomas
The Center For New Life
3251 Brookview Dr.
Casper, Wyoming 82604
(307) 237-9676

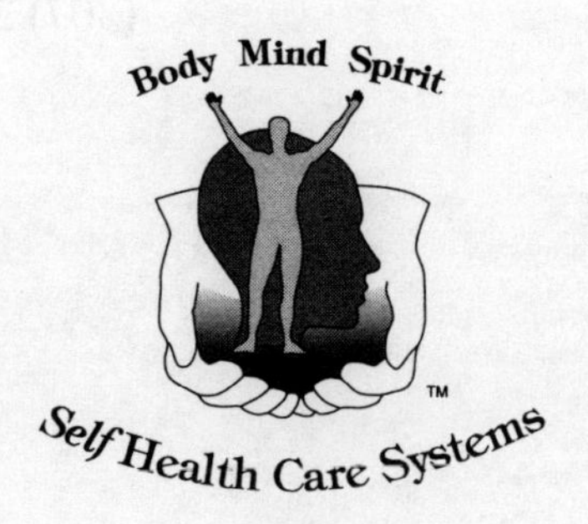
Body Mind Spirit
TM
Self Health Care Systems

Bibliography

Abramowski O. L. M., M.D. *Fruitarian Healing System*. Natal, South Africa: Essence of Health, 1976.

Alberts, Bruce, and Dennis Bray, Julian Lewis *et. al. Molecular Biology of The Cell*, 3rd edition. New York: Garland Publishing Co., 1983.

Alcott, William A. *The Teacher of Health and the Laws of the Human Constitution*. Boston: D. S. King and Co., 1843.

Allen, Hannah. *Fasting: Fastest Way to Superb Health and Rejuvenation*. Austin, Texas: Life Science Society (publication not dated).

------------. "Why We Should Not Eat Animal Product in Any Form." *Life Science Health System, Lesson #33* by T.C. Fry. Austin, Texas: Life Science, 1983.

------------. "Why We Should Not Eat Meat." *Life Science Health System, Lesson #32* by T.C. Fry. Austin, Texas: Life Science, 1983.

Altman, Nathaniel. *Eating For Life*. Wheaton, Illinois: Theosophical Publishers, 1974.

Andrews, Arthur D. *Eat Your Way To Glowing Health*. Affton, Missouri: Good Life Publications, 1957.

Annand, J.C. "Further Evidence in the Case Against Heated Milk Protein, Atherosclerosis." *Journal of the College of General Practitioners*, Vol. 7, 1964.

Atkinson, Donald T. *Myth, Magic and Medicine*. Cleveland: World Publishing Co., 1956.

Bach, Edward. *Heal Thyself*. London: Daniel, 1946.

Baron, Samuel, M.D. *Medical Microbiology*. Menlo Park, California: Addison-Hensley Publishing Co., 1982.

Bauman, Edward, *et al*. *The Holistic Health Handbook*. Berkeley, California; And/Or Press, 1978.

Bealle, Morris A. *The Drug Story*. Spanish Fork, Utah: The Hornet's Nest, 1949.

------------. *The New Drug Story*. Washington, D.C.: Columbia Publishing Co., 1958.

Bear, John, Ph.D. *Bear's Guide to Non-Traditional College Degrees*, 9th edition. Berkeley, California: Ten Speed Press, 1985.

Beck, Melinda. "Health Care: Painful Remedies." *Newsweek*. March 1, 1993.

------------. "Doctors Under the Knife." *Newsweek*. April 5, 1993.

Beiler, Henry G. *Food Is Your Best Medicine*. New York: Random House, 1965.

Bell, G. *Textbook of Physiology and Biochemistry*, 4th edit. Baltimore, Ohio: Williams and Wilkins, 1959.

Bernard, Raymond W. *Are You Being Poisoned By the Foods You Eat?* Mokelhumme Hill, California: Health Research, 1956.

------------. *Eat Your Way To Better Health*, Vol I & II. Clarksburg, West Virginia: Saucerian, 1974.

Bidwell, Victoria. "Lesson #21: Natural Weight-Loss Systems" *Life Science Health System* by T .C. Fry. Austin, Texas: Life Science, 1983.

Bircher-Benner, M. *Eating Your Way To Better Health*. Baltimore, Maryland: Penguin, 1973.

Bisset, Kenneth A. *The Cytology and Life History of Bacteria* Edinburgh, Pennsylvania: Livingstone, 1970.

Blakiston's Pocket Medical Dictionary. New York: McGraw-Hill Book Co., 1979.

Bordley, James. *Two Centuries of American Medicine*. Philadelphia: Saunders, 1976.

Bricklin, Mark. *The Practical Encyclopedia of Natural Healing*. Emmaus, Pennsylvania: Rodale Press, 1976.

Brieger, Gert H. *Medical America in the 19th Century*. Baltimore, Maryland: John Hopkins Press, 1972.

Brown, Richard E. *Rockefeller Medicine Men: Medicine and Capitalism in America* . Berkeley, California: University of California Press, 1979.

Bureau of the Census; and Economics and Statistics Administration, U .S. Department of Commerce. *Statistical Abstract of the United States: 1992* . Washington D.C.: U.S. Government Printing Office, 1992.

Burkitt, Denis P., F.R.C.S., F.R.C. "Some Diseases Characterstics of Modern Western Civilization." *British Medical Journal* , Vol. 1, February 1973.

Burnett, Frank M. *The Virus and the Cell* . Washington D.C.: U.S. Government Printing Office, 1953.

Campbell, T. Colin, Ph.D. "Diet and Disease: The China Study". Excerpts from 1991 AHNS Conference lecture, prepared by Hope Gray, Susan Taylor and James Lennon. *Health Science* Tampa, Florida: American Natural Hygiene Society, September / October 1992.

Cancer Facts and Figures . American Cancer Society, 1983.

"Can Fruit Help You Lose Weight?" *Bergen Record* , October 20, 1983.

Carey, George W., M.D. *The Chemistry Wonders of the Human Body* . Mokelhumme Hill, California; Health Research, 1921.

Carque, Otto. *Vital Facts About Foods* . New Canaan, Connecticut: Keats, 1975.

Carrington, Hereward, Ph.D. *Fasting For Health and Long Life* 1st edition. Mokelhumme Hill, California: Health Research, 1908.

------------. *The History of Natural Hygiene* . Mokelhumme Hill, California: Health Research, 1964.

------------. *The Natural Food of Man* . Mokelhumme Hill, California: Health Research, 1963.

Cassedy, James H. *Medicine in America: A Short History* . Baltimore, Maryland: John Hopkins University Press, 1991.

Castro, Janice. "Paging Dr. Clinton". *Time* . January 18, 1993.

Chen, Edwin. "Lid on Health Care Costs Needed, Gore Says". *Los Angeles Times* , March 30, 1993.

------------. "New Payroll Deduction May Fund Health Plan". *Los Angeles Times* , May 1, 1993.

------------. "Payroll Levy Idea in Health Plan Detailed." *Los Angeles Times* , May 7, 1993.

Cheraskin, Emanual, M.D., W. Ringsdorf, M.D., and J.H. Clark. *Diet and Disease* Emmaus, Pennsylvania: Rodale Press, 1968.

Chopra, Deepak, M.D. *Quantum Healing* . New York: Bantam Books, 1989.

Cinque, Ralph C., D.C. "Hygiene v.s. Therapy." *Health Science* Tampa, Florida: American Natural Hygiene Society, March-April 1993.

Clements, George Ph.D., and Shelton, Herbert M., Ph.D. *Elementary Orthopathy: Teaching a New Science of Health and Natural Healing* . Mokelhumme Hill, California: Health Research, 1963.

Clift, Eleanor. "Hillary's Hard Sell." *Newsweek* . March 29, 1993.

Clifton, Charles E. *An Introduction To Bacterial Physiology* . New York: McGraw Hill, 1957.

Committee of Diet, Nutrition and Cancer: Assembly of Life Sciences National Research Council. *Diet Nutrition and Cancer* . Washington, D.C.: National Academy Press, 1982.

Consumer Reports. *The New Medicine Show* , 6th edition. Mount Vernon, New York: Consumers Union of the United States, 1989.

------------. "Wasted Health Care Dollars." *Consumer Reports.* Mount Vernon, New York: Consumers Union of the United States, July 1992.

Cornett, Frederick D., and Pauline Gratz. *Modern Human Physiology* . New York: Holt, Rinehart and Winston, 1982.

Cousins, Norman. *Anatomy of an Illness* . New York: Bantam Books, 1979.

D'Adamo, Janus, M.D. *One Man's Food* . New York: Richard Marek, 1980.

Densmore, Emmet, M.D. *How Nature Cures* . Mokelhumme Hill, California: Health Research, 1892.

Diamond, Harvey, and Marilyn Diamond. *Fit For Life* . New York: Warner Books, 1985.

------------. *Fit For Life II: Living Health, The Complete Health Program* . New York: Warner Books, 1988.

------------. "Highlights From Fit For Life Talk, 1992 ANHS Conference, Washington D.C." *American Natural Hygiene Society cassette*. Tampa, Florida: American Natural Hygiene Society, 1992.

Dougherty, A. "Ethical Values in Health Care Reform." *The Journal of the American Medical Association*. November 4, 1992.

Dubos, Rene, J. *The Bacterial Cell in Its Relation to Problems of Virulence, Immunity and Chemotherapy*. Cambridge, Massachusetts: Harvard University Press, 1945.

Eckert, John, and David Randall. *Animal Physiology: Mechanisms and Adaptation*, 2nd edition. New York: W.H. Freeman and Co., 1983.

Ehret, Arnold. *Mucusless Diet Healthing System*. New York: Benedict Lust, 1976.

Esser, William L. *Dictionary of Man's Foods*. Chicago: Natural Hygiene Press, 1972.

Farb, Peter, and George Armelagos. *The Anthropology of Eating* Boston: Houghton Miffin Co., 1980.

Fathman, George, and Doris Fathman. *Live Foods*. Beaumont, California: Ehret Literature Publishing, 1973.

Fleming, Donald. *William H. Welch and the Rise of Modern Medicine*. Boston: Little Brown, 1954.

Flexner, Abraham. *Funds and Foundations: Their Policies, Past and Present*. New York: Harper, 1952.

------------. *I Remember: The Autobiography of Abraham Flexner*. New York: Simon & Schuster, 1940.

Fraenkel-Conrat, Heinz. *The Chemistry and Biology of Viruses* New York: Academic Press, 1969.

Fraser, Dean. *Viruses and Molecular Biology*. New York: MacMillan, 1967.

Freymann, John G. *The American Health Care System: Its Genesis and Trajectory*. Huntington, New York: R.E. Krieger Publishing Co., 1977.

Fruits. Alexandria, Virginia: Time-Life Books, 1983.

Fry, T.C. *The Great AIDS Hoax*, 3rd edition. Manchaca, Texas: Health Excellence Systems, 1989.

------------. *High Energy Methods, Lessons #1-7*. Austin, Texas: Life Science, 1983.

------------. *The Life Science Health System, Lessons #1-111.* Austin, Texas: Life Science, 1983.

------------. *The Myth of Medicine* . Austin, Texas: Life Science, 1974.

------------. *The Revelation of Health* . Austin, Texas: Life Science, 1981.

------------. *Super Food For Super Health* . Austin, Texas: Life Science, 1976.

------------. *Superior Foods, Diet Principles and Practices For Perfect Health* . Austin, Texas: Life Science, 1974.

------------. *The Ultimate Diet: Superior Foods, Diet Principles and Practices For Perfect Health* . Austin, Texas: Life Science (publication not dated).

Glaser, Ronald. *The Body is the Hero* . New York: Random House, 1976.

Goldhammer, Alan, D.C. "Natural Hygiene: The Science of Health." *Healthful Living* . Austin, Texas: Life Science, November/December 1989.

Gore, Rick. "The Awesome Worlds Within a Cell." *National Geographic* . March 1976.

Graham, Sylvester, *et .al* . *The Greatest Health Discovery* . Chicago: Natural Hygiene press, 1972.

------------. *Lectures on the Science of Human Life* . Mokelhumme Hill, California: Health Research, 1883.

Gray, Henry, M.D. *Gray's Anatomy* . New York: Bounty Books, 1977.

Greenberg, Daniel S. "Change in Course for Health Insurance Industry." *The Lancet* . December 12, 1992.

Guyton, Arthur C. *Guidance Textbook of Medical Physiology* . Philadelphia: Saunders Publishing Co., 1981.

------------. *Physiology of the Body* . Philadelphia: W.B. Saunders, 1981.

------------. *Physiology of the Human Body* . Philadelphia: Saunders College Publishing, 1984.

"Heart Facts" . American Heart Association, 1984.

Henrici, Arthur T. *The Biology of Bacteria: An Introduction to General Microbiology* , 3rd edition. Boston: D.C. Heath, 1948.

Hiatt, Don. "Can Medical Care Be Called Health Care?" *Health Freedom News.* National Health Federation: Monrovia, California, October 1992.

Horne, Robert W. *The Structure and Function of Viruses*. London: E. Arnold, 1978.

Hotema, Hilton. *Perfect Health*. Natal, South Africa: Essence of Health, (publication not dated).

Hovannessian, A.T. *Raw Eating*. Tehran: Arshavir, 1967.

Howell, W.H., M.D. *The Human Machine*. Ontario, Canada: Provoker Press, 1969.

Hume, E. Douglas. *Be'champ or Pasteur? A Lost Chapter in the History of Biology*. Rochford, England: C.W. Daniel, 1947.

Hunter, Beatrice T. *Consumer Beware: Your Food and What's Been Done to It*.New York: Simon & Schuster, 1972.

Illich, Ivan. *Medical Nemesis*. New York: Bantam, 1976.

Keeton, William T. *Biological Science*, 3rd edition. New York: W.W. Norton and Co., 1980.

Knight, Claude Arthur. *Chemistry of Viruses*. Wien, Springer. 1963.

Koch, Robert. *Essays of Robert Koch translated by K. Codell Carter*. New York: Greenwood Press, 1987.

Kogan, Benjamin A., Ph.D. *Health: Man In A Changing Environment*. New York: Harcourt, Bruce and World Inc., 1970.

Krok, Morris. *Amazing New Health System*. Natal, South Africa: Essence of Health, 1976.

------------. *Formula For Long Life*. Natal, South Africa: Essence of Health, 1977.

------------. *Fruit, The Food and Medicine For Man*. Natal, South Africa: Essence of Health, 1967.

------------. *Health Truths Eternal*. Natal, South Africa: Essence of Health, 1964.

Kugler, Hans, J. Ph.D. *et. al*. "Special Issue: The Health Care Crisis." Vol. 5. *Preventive Medicine Update*. International Academy of Holistic Health and Medicine. Redondo Beach, California: 1992

Lauter, David. "First Lady Issues Warning on Health Care" *Los Angeles Times,* April 17, 1993.

------------. "Rising Health Care Costs May Erase Cuts in Deficit." *Los Angeles Times*, April 9, 1993.

Levy, Hilton, B. *The Biochemistry of Viruses*. New York: M. Decker, 1969.

Lewin, Benjamin. *Genes*, 2nd edition. New York: John Wiley and Sons, 1985.

Linkswiler, Helen M. *Nutrition Review's Present Knowledge in Nutrition*, 4th edition. New York: The Nutrition Foundation, 1976.

Lohnis, F. *Studies Upon the Lifecycles of Bacteria*. National Academy of Sciences, Washington D.C.: U.S. Government Printing Office, 1921.

Longwood, William. *Poisons in Your Food*. New York: Pyramid, 1969.

Luce, Gay Goar, Ph.D. *Body Time: Physiological Rhythms*. New York: Pantheon, 1971.

Marks, Geoffrey. *The Story of Medicine in America*. New York: Scribner, 1973.

Mendelsohn, Robert S., M.D. *Confessions of a Medical Heretic* New York: Warner Books, 1980.

Metchnikoff, Elie. *The Founders of Modern Medicine: Pasteur, Koch, Lister*. New York: Walden Publications, 1979.

Mizrahi, Terry. "Chaotic and Costly Health Care Scene." National Health Line, *Health and Social Work*. August 1992.

Moffat, Susan. "Brothers Face Charges of $1-Billion Fraud." *Los Angeles Times*, March 16, 1993.

Moore-Ede, Martin C. *The Clocks That Time Us*. Boston, Massachusetts: Harvard University Press, 1982.

Morbidity and Mortality Weekly Report. Center For Disease Control, Atlanta.

Mullins, Eustace. *Murder By Injection: The Story of the Medical Conspiracy Against America*. Staunton, Virginia: The National Council for Medical Research, 1988.

Munro, Ian R. M.D. "How Not to Improve Health Care." *Readers Digest*, September 1992.

National Geographic Society. *The Incredible Machine*. Washington, D.C.: National Geographic Society, 1986.

Nicol, Hugh. *Microbes By the Million*. Harmondsworth, Middlesex England: Penguin Books limited, 1939.

Nolfi, Cristine, M.D. *My Experiences With Living Food*. Ontario, Canada: Provoker Press, 1969.

"Nutrition and Health." *Nutrition Health Review #37.* January 1986.

Oldfield, Josiah, Ph.D *Eat Nature's Food and Live Long*. Mokelhumme Hill, California: Health Research, 1960.

Park, William H.*Who's Who Among the Microbes*. New York: Century Co., 1929.

Page, Melvin, and H.L. Abrams. *Your Body Is Your Best Doctor* New Canaan, Connecticut: Keats, 1972.

Pearson, R.B. *Pasteur: Plagiarist, Imposter*. Mokelhumme Hill, California: Health Research, 1942.

The Progressive. Comment "Inappropriate Remedies." *The Progressive*. November 1992.

Prosser, C. *Comparative Animal Physiology*, 2nd edition. St. Louis: W.B. Saunders, 1961.

Rahn, Otto. *Microbes of Merit*. Lancaster, Pennsylvania: The Jacques Cattell Press, 1945.

Ray P, and Gupta, H.N. *Caraka Samhita*. Calcutta, India: Sree Saraswaty Press, 1965.

Resnick, Charlotte A., and Gloria R. Resnick. *To Your Good Health*. New York: Amsco School Publications Inc., 1979.

Reuben, David, M.D. *Everything You Always Wanted To Know About Nutrition*. New York: Avon, 1979.

Robinson, Victor. *The Story of Medicine*. New York: The New Home Library, 1943.

Saunders, David S. *An Introduction To Biological Rhythms*. New York: Wiley, 1977.

Select Committee on Nutrition and Human Needs, U.S. Senate. *Dietary Goals for the United States*. Washington D.C.: U.S. Government Printing Office, 977.

Shelton, Herbert M., Ph.D. "Are Humans Meat Eaters?" *The Life Science Health System, Lesson #88*. Austin, Texas: Life Science, 1983.

------------. *Dr. Shelton's Hygienic Review*, Vols. I through V Mokelhumme Hill, California; Health Research, September 1939 through August 1944.
------------. *Fasting Can Save Your Life*. Chicago: Natural Hygiene Press, 1964.
------------. *Food Combining Made Easy*. San Antonio, Texas Dr. Shelton's Health School, 1951.
------------. *Getting Well*. Mokelhumme Hill, California: Health Research, (publication not dated).
------------. *Health For All*. Mokelhumme Hill, California: Health Research, (publication not dated).
------------. *Human Beauty, Its Culture and Hygiene*. San Antonio, Texas: Dr. Shelton's Health School, 1934.
------------. *Human Life: Its Philosophy and Laws*. Mokelhumme Hill, California: Health Research, 1979.
------------. *The Hygienic System*, Vol I, II & III. San Antonio, Texas: Dr. Shelton's Health School, 1964.
------------. *Natural Hygiene, Man's Pristine Way of Life*. San Antonio, Texas; Dr. Shelton's Health School, 1964.
------------. *Orthobionomics—Vol I of the Hygienic System* Mokelhumme Hill, California: Health Research, 1934.
------------. *Principles of Natural Hygiene*. San Antonio, Texas: Dr. Shelton's Health School, 1964.
------------. *The Science and Fine Art of Fasting*. Chicago: Natural Hygiene Press, 1978.
------------. *Superior Nutrition*. San Antonio, Texas: Dr. Shelton's Health School, 1951.
Sherman, Henry C., M.D. *Essentials of Nutrition*, 4th edition. New York: MacMillian, 1957.
Sherman, Irwin W., and Vilia G. Sherman.*Biology: A Human Approach*, 2nd edition. New York: Oxford University Press, 1979.
Shuit, Douglas P. "Survey Finds Public Highly Insecure About Health Care." *Los Angeles Times*, April 9, 1993.
Smith, Kenneth M. *The Biology of Viruses*. London: Oxford University Press, 1965.
Smith, Lee. "The Right Cure for Health Care." *Fortune*. October 19, 1992.

Spencer, R.P. *The Intestinal Tract*. Springfield, Illinois: Charles Thomas Publishers, 1960.

Stanley, W. Jacob, M.D., Clarice A. Francone, and Walter J. Lessow, Ph.D. *Structure and Function in Man*, 5th edition. Philadelphia: W.B. Saunders Co. 1982.

Thimann, Kenneth. *The Life of Bacteria: Their Growth, Metabolism and Relationships*. New York: MacMillan, 1963.

Tilden, John H., M.D. *Food: Its Composition, Preparation, and Combination*. Denver: J.H. Tilden, 1916.

------------. *Toxemia Explained*. Denver, Colorado: Health Research, 1926.

Tootill, Elizabeth. *The Facts on File: Dictionary of Biology*. New York: Facts On File Inc., 1981.

Trall, Russell T., M.D. *The Hydropathic Encyclopedia*. New York: Fowlers and Wells, 1854.

----------- *The Hygienic System*. Battle Creek, Michigan: The Office of the Health Reformer, 1872.

------------. *Popular Physiology*. Mokelhumme Hill, California: Health Research, 1884.

------------. *The True Healing Art, Hygiene vs. Drug Medication*, an address delivered in the Smithsonian Institute. Washington D.C. Mokelhumme Hill, California: Health Research, 1880.

Trop, Jack D. *You Don't Have To Be Sick*. New York: Julian Press, 1961.

Tufts University Diet and Nutrition Letter *"Doctors Fail To Make the Nutritional Grade."* New York: Tufts University, April 1993.

Upton, Arthur C., M.D., Director National Cancer Institute. *Statement on the Status of the Diet, Nutrition and Cancer Program*, before the Subcommittee on Nutrition. Senate Committee on Agriculture, Nutrition and Forestry, October 2, 1972.

Verrett, Jacqueline, and Jean Carper. *Eating May Be Hazardous To Your Health*. New York: Simon & Schuster, 1974.

Waerland, Are. *Health Is Your Birthright*. Bern, Switzerland Humata Publishers, *Circa* 1945.

Walker, Alan, Ph.D. "Research Yields Surprises About Early Human Diets." *New York Times*, May 15, 1979.

Walker, N.W., D.Sc. *Become Younger*. Phoenix, Arizona: Norwalk Press, 1949.

------------. *Natural Weight Control*. Phoenix, Arizona: O'Sullivan Woodside and Co., 1981.

------------. *Vibrant Health*. Phoenix, Arizona: O'Sullivan Woodside and Co., 1972.

Weger, George S., Herbert M. Shelton, T.C. Fry *et al*. *How To Keep Your Body Pure*. Austin, Texas: Life Science, (publication not dated).

Weiss, Stefanie. "Health Care Crisis: Finally, Some Action." *NEA Today* February 1992.

Whiteman-Jones, Michael. "Clinton & Health Care Reform." *Delicious!* April 1993

Wigmore, Ann. *Be Your Own Doctor*. Boston: Hippocrates Health Institute, 1973.

Winter, Ruth. *Beware of the Food You Eat*. New York: Signet, 1971.

Woolsey, Raymond H. *Meat on the Menu, Who Needs It?* Washington D.C.: Review and Herald Publishing, 1974.

Wynder, E. "The Dietary Environment and Cancer." *Journal of the American Dietetic Association*, Vol. 71, 1977.

Yerushamy, J., Ph.D., and Herman E. Hilleboe, M.D. "Fat in the Diet and Mortality from Heart Disease." *New York State Journal of Medicine*, Vol. 57, July 15, 1957.

Yudkin John, M.D. *Sweet and Dangerous*. New York:Bantam, 1972.

Index

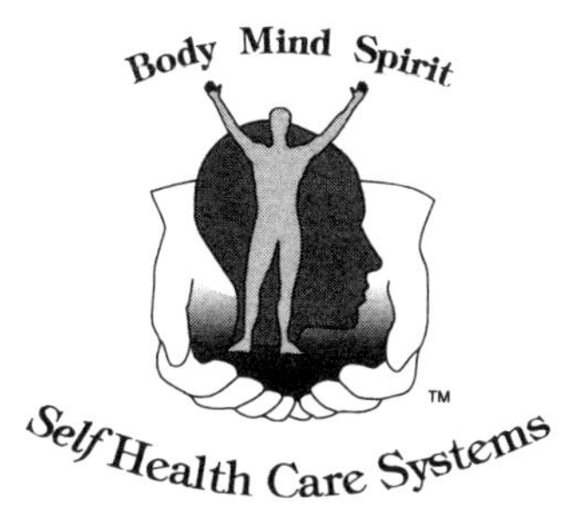
Body Mind Spirit
TM
Self Health Care Systems